Swedish Massage

with
Dr. James Mally

Ninth Printing 2017
Eighth Printing 2012
Seventh Printing 2009
Sixth Printing 2007
Fifth Printing 2005
Fourth Printing 2003
Third Printing 2002
Second Printing 2001
First Printing 2000

ISBN Numbers:
0-9666533-5-1   Swedish Massage Workbook
0-9721380-0-5   Swedish Massage DVD
0-9666533-6-X   Swedish Massage DVD and Workbook

Table of Contents

This workbook is designed to complement the Swedish Massage DVD and to aid in learning the individual techniques. The techniques are grouped into routines both for ease of learning and ease of practice. The techniques are organized in a way that is logical and that flows well from one technique to another. The routines are like containers to hold the strokes, but the order in the routines should not be taken as gospel. If you find other techniques or different routines that work for you, that is fine.

Some therapists prefer to not use routines but to work totally by intuition. The down side of that approach is that it is possible to miss muscle groups or even whole parts of the body. It can be embarrassing when you finish a massage to have a client ask, "Are you going to massage my right leg?" A routine can insure that all areas are covered in a massage.

The downside of using a routine is that the massage may seem too ordered and predictable and may lack a sense of the client's needs in the moment. When a routine is mastered, it frees you from having to figure out what you are going to do next. In this freedom you can deviate from the routine to work longer in areas that are tight and to use extra or different strokes where needed. This approach frees you so that you are able to use your intuition in an effective way. To keep your massage from feeling predictable, it is possible to have several different routines that you use, and to frequently deviate from those routines as your intuition suggests.

In the beginning, students often take 1 1/2 to 2 hours to complete a full body massage. This is because they will often do the same stroke 20 times while trying to figure out what to do next. Not only is this not efficient, but it gets very tiring to the client as they are waiting for you to move on to something else. When tight areas are found you can work longer, however, if you work too long in one area, it can be irritating to your client. It is better to work for shorter amounts of time in an area, leave and come back to the area later. With a routine you can flow from one stoke to the next, to the next, performing each stroke just 3 or 4 times. Massage initiates the healing through stimulating the nervous system and the circulation, but much healing happens even after our hands have left the area. You may be surprised how much an area can relax when you let it be after massaging it.

Sometimes students with a good intuitive grasp of massage go through a period of frustration when learning new techniques. Because of the left brain focus on learning the new techniques, they feel they lose their flow and intuitive sense. This is temporary and once they have mastered the new techniques they find their flow and intuition returning so they can give an even better massage.

Massage is balancing for the therapist as well as the client. It balances the left and right sides of your body because whatever you do on one side of your client you repeat on the other side. It also balances between the left and right sides of the brain. The left brain understanding of anatomy can enhance the intuition of the right brain. One way I like to do this is by visualizing the layers of muscles underneath your hands while you work. Doing this enhances your intuitive sense of the muscles. As you find a balance between intellect and intuition you will become much more effective in your massage.

Whether you are using this DVD and workbook to learn massage for the first time, or to add to what you already know, I hope you enjoy what you learn here.

Index

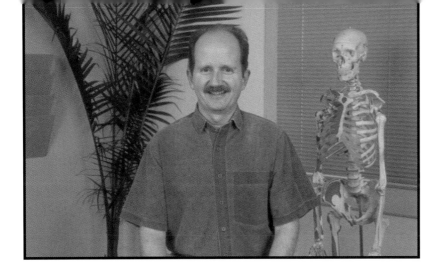

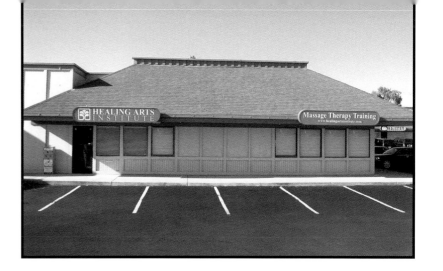

Dr. James Mally has been doing massage professionally in many different settings since 1975. He is a graduate of both the John Bastyr College of Naturopathic Medicine, a four-year accredited medical school covering all aspects of natural therapeutics and the Lindsey Hopkins School, a 1000-hour massage training program. Dr. Mally is able to integrate his thorough knowledge of anatomy and physiology with the practice of massage. He has been teaching massage certification programs since 1979, and is currently teaching advanced classes in deep tissue massage, sports massage, and applied anatomy in massage schools around the country.

Healing Arts Institute is located in Citrus Heights, California, a suburb of Sacramento. The institute offers state certified trainings in therapeutic massage and acupressure massage as well as advanced classes in deep tissue massage, sports massage, geriatric massage, reflexology, and many other bodywork related subjects.

The relaxed atmosphere of this setting helps to create a supportive learning environment. Our advanced workshops and three-week massage intensives attract students from all over the world. For information about classes call us at 916-725-3999, or visit us on the web at:

www.healingartsinstitute.com

Glossary

Abduct – to draw away from the midline

Adduct – to draw back toward the midline

Adductors – a muscle group in the medial thigh that adducts the leg

Anterior – toward the front of the body

ASIS – Anterior Superior Iliac Spine - the front of the crest of the hip

Axilla – armpit

Circumduction – a cone shaped movement

Deltoid – triangular shaped muscle over the top of the shoulder

Distal – further away from the torso

Effleurage – a gliding stroke

Erector Spinae – postural muscles on either side of the spine

Fulling – a heel press - pressing with the heels of your hands moving away from each other

Gastrocnemius – superficial muscle on the back of the calf

Greater Trochanter – the part of the proximal femur (thigh bone) that sticks out laterally

Iliac Crest – the crest of the ilium (upper part of the pelvis)

Inferior – going toward the feet, below

Intercostal – in between the ribs

Ischium – one of the bones of the pelvis, the one you sit on

Lateral – moving away from the midline

Levator Scapulae – a muscle in the back of the neck that raises the scapula

Lordosis – an anterior (forward) curve of the spine

Mastoid Process – a bony projection of the temporal bone - just behind the ear

Medial – toward the midline

Occiput – occipital bone - base of the skull

Petrissage – kneading

Popliteal – the area behind the knee

Posterior – towards the back of the body

Prone – lying face down

Proximal – toward the torso

Sacrum – triangular shaped bone at the base of the spine

Scapula – shoulder blade

Soleus – deep muscle on the back of the calf

Spinous Process – the part of a vertebrae that projects posteriorly

Sternocleidomastoid – a muscle on the front of the neck

Sternum – breastbone

Superior – towards the head

Supine – lying face up

Supraspinatus – a muscle on the superior part of the scapula

Tapotement – percussion

Transverse Processes – the parts of a vertebrae that project laterally

Xyphoid Process – the inferior tip of the sternum

Zygomatic Arch – the cheekbone

Body Mechanics

If you work bending over and are using your upper body excessively you may develop back pain and problems through your shoulders and arms. It is very important while giving a massage to keep your back straight and to move from your center. The preferred movement to practice is a lunge in which the power comes from your legs and the power is directed by your arms and hands. You can work long hours and not get fatigued by working this way.

When you use your body in ways you are not accustomed to, you may experience some discomfort at first. This may be the natural discomfort of doing something new or different, in which case the discomfort should ease as the movements become familiar. Please keep practicing, paying attention to your body mechanics, your breathing, your client and their response. Have another massage therapist observe the DVD and observe you practicing while watching your body mechanics. They may see something in the way you move that you aren't aware of.

If a technique still feels uncomfortable after repeated practice, it's possible that it may not be suited either to your body type or for the particular client you are practicing on. You may need to vary the technique to have it feel comfortable, or you may need to abandon it altogether.

If you notice any aches or pains developing, pay close attention to your body mechanics as you work. You may find certain movements or techniques cause or aggravate your pain. I once had wrist pain that was caused by a particular stroke that I was taught. Once I modified that stroke the wrist pain subsided and I've had no more problems with it.

Attitude also plays a part in how your body handles the stresses of an activity. If you enjoy what you are doing you are less likely to suffer a repetitive stress injury than if you dislike it. Your feelings affect your muscle tension and the stress on your joints. Fortunately, giving a massage is enjoyable work. If you should start to feel burned out doing massage, get a massage yourself so you can be rejuvenated and reminded of the good you do. Taking workshops and learning different techniques can help as well.

History of Swedish Massage

Massage has been practiced in many cultures for as long as people have been around. Cave paintings in Europe show it in use around 15,000 B.C., and most ancient cultures had a tradition of massage. Massage was used by the Egyptians, the Romans, and the ancient Greeks. Hippocrates (460 - 375 B.C.), considered the father of western medicine, had a great respect for the effectiveness of massage. He is quoted as saying "the physician must be skilled in many things and particularly friction."

Although massage is as old as mankind, Swedish massage has a much more recent history. It was developed by Pehr Henrik Ling (1776 - 1839) in Sweden, incorporating medical gymnastics, active, passive and resisted movements, long gliding strokes, kneading and friction. It became very popular in Europe then came to the United States in the mid 1800's. In the US it was promoted and popularized by people such as John Harvey Kellogg (1852 - 1943) with his sanitarium at Battle Creek, Michigan, and Douglas O. Graham. Unfortunately, Kellogg and Graham are now remembered more for corn flakes and graham crackers, both originally health foods before sugar was added.

Massage went through a decline in the mid 20th century because of the rise of technological medicine, but it has been showing a strong resurgence since the 1980s as people have been looking for a more human and practical approach to healing.

Many different types of bodywork have been developed that complement, and can be integrated with, Swedish Massage. Esalen massage, developed at the Esalen Institute in Big Sur, California, is a slower, more rhythmic massage designed to facilitate a deeper state of relaxation. Reflexology uses pressure on points in the feet, hands or ears to affect the various organs and systems of the body to promote health. Trigger point therapy is used to release tension in specific areas of the body. Deep Tissue Massage works slowly and deeply to work out deeper layers of tension in the muscles and fascia. Sports massage aids an athlete in recovery or rehabilitation after an injury or event, and can be used to improve athletic performance. These techniques, and many more, may be blended with Swedish massage techniques to give a massage that best meets the needs of an individual client.

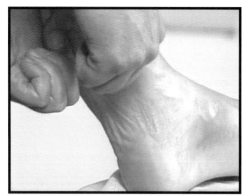
1. Working into arch with fingers

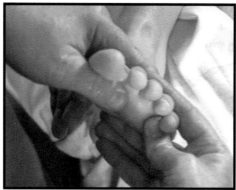
2. Thumbands into metatarsal space

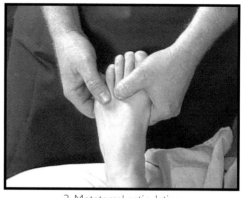
3. Metatarsal articulation

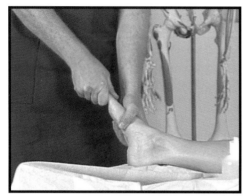
4. Toe articulation and pull

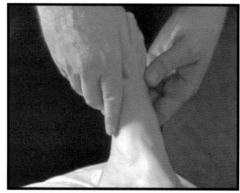
5. Tendon Grooves on dorsal surface

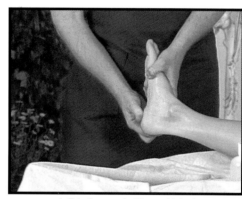
6. Friction to Ankle and Heel

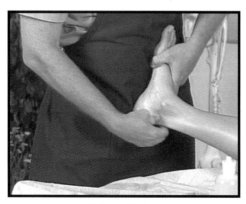
7. Dorsiflexion

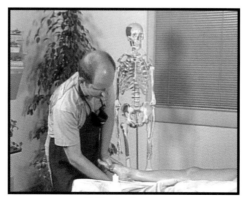
8. Plantarflexion

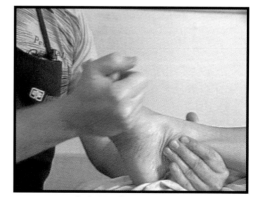
9. Ankle Circumduction

Basic Massage Strokes

EFFLEURAGE: The principle Swedish massage stroke. It consists of a gliding motion using the full flat surface of the hand and fingers which gently mold and conform to the body. Pressure may be light to produce a relaxing and sedative effect. Pressure may be increased, keeping the hand relaxed and supple to maximize venous and lymphatic return. Especially applicable for initial oiling, effleurage is also a connecting stroke that can be used between more vigorous strokes, providing a sense of continuity and relaxation. When performed with moderate pressure, effleurage should be directed towards the heart, preventing damage to delicate valves and promoting proper circulation. Effleurage is uniquely sedative and enjoyable when carried out slowly and steadily. Effleurage feels best when the full length of the muscle is stroked from one end to the other.

PETRISSAGE: A firm kneading and compressing of muscular and subcutaneous tissues. A variety of techniques such as pinching, plucking, squeezing, folding, lifting and rolling are all included in this category. The hands should be pliable but firm, as in the working of dough. Petrissage aids circulation by dilating blood vessels, and reduces muscle spasm by breaking up adhesions or densely bunched connective tissue. The increased circulation causes waste products to be eliminated from the tissues more quickly. Petrissage is an excellent form of passive exercise and is an aid to maintaining skin tone and elasticity. Petrissage should be executed fairly vigorously but never to the point of inducing pain. The client should experience an increased sense of relaxation and vitality as circulation and balance is restored to the area.

FRICTION: Friction is defined as any stroke of moderate to firm pressure that repeatedly crosses the grain of a muscle or muscle group, or any stroke of sufficient contact and movement as to generate heat in the tissues. Friction can be performed in a variety of ways, adapting to the size and shape of each body part. Friction can be "spot specific" or moving over a more general area. Examples:

"Superficial Friction" - Rapid movement of the hands over the skin.

"Deep Friction" - A rapid movement of the palm with full stationary contact to the skin, or minimal gliding over the skin's surface, so that the skin is moved over underlying tissues.

"Circular Friction" - A rapid circular movement of the palm with either full stationary contact to the skin (deep circular friction), or gliding over the skin's surface (superficial circular friction).

"Scrubbing" - Repeated vigorous strokes using the flat side of the knuckles or an alternating "push-pull" motion in one area using hands, knuckles, or forearms, which generates heat in the tissues.

"Fulling or Heel-press" - A broad flat pressure across a larger area such as the low back, usually performed slowly and steadily with the full hand, emphasis of pressure on the heel.

"Thumb-bands" - A very specific pulling across the grain of a muscle, or muscle group such as the erector spinae muscles. The thumbs work simultaneously pulling in opposing directions.

Primary benefits of friction are: dilating capillary beds, stimulating venous and lymph circulation, stripping trapped toxins in tissues, stretching, opening and "unbunching" dense or congested muscle tissue, reducing muscular spasm and increasing warmth in the treated area. Friction can be very invigorating and is especially appropriate before and after athletic competition. Care should be taken that friction is not applied to raw, broken or overly sensitive skin.

TAPOTEMENT (Percussion): Any series of rhythmical impacts upon the body that send a wave-like vibration into underlying tissues and organs. The quality and intensity of the vibration is varied by the positioning of the hands. Specific techniques include: hacking, cupping, slapping, tapping, and light pounding. Percussion is generally very stimulating. The effects of percussion can be quite pronounced on internal organs such as the lungs, adrenals, kidneys or pancreas, and care must be taken, especially over the kidneys, to use only light impacts. Care should be taken not to over-stimulate especially in an ill or debilitated client. Percussion should not be used on any area where a fracture is suspected. Percussion and postural drainage is an effective way to relieve lung congestion when performed properly.

Primary benefits of percussion are in its stimulating effect on the skin, subcutaneous, vascular, and muscular tissue and on the underlying organs. Prolonged heavy percussion along a muscle group may produce numbness or apparent anesthesia due to fatigue of the nerve endings. This technique can be useful therefore in releasing an area of chronic muscular tension and providing significant pain relief.

JOINT ARTICULATION: Joint Articulation is the movement of a joint through its normal range of motion. Movement to a joint is accomplished by bending, rotating, or circumducting the adjacent bone. Generally the more proximal portion of the body part is stabilized as the more distal portion is mobilized. In larger joints such as the hip, this stabilization is provided by body weight. In all joint articulation the client remains passive, allowing the full weight of the body part to be supported by the therapist, as the joint is moved to the limit of its normal range of motion. If a joint is stiff, inflamed or otherwise painful, great care should be taken to stay well within the client's comfort level. Increasing the range of motion can be done gradually over a series of treatments. Primary benefits of joint articulation include; increasing to normal range of motion and preventing limitation or degeneration of the joint due to a thickening and reduced efficiency of the synovial fluid.

Leg Strokes Supine Sequence

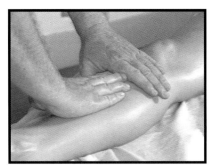

1. Long Stroke

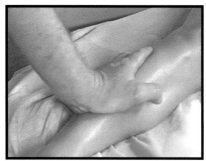

2. Tibialis Side Stretch

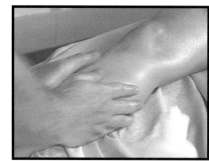

3. Heels up Tibia

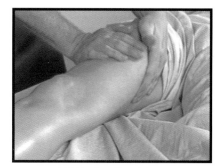

4. Wringing Quadriceps

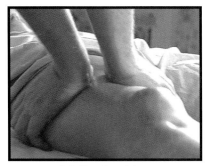

5. Fulling Quadriceps

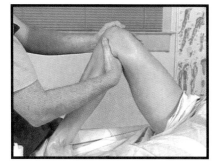

6. Popliteal Tendon Stretch

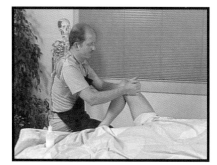

7. Working around Knee

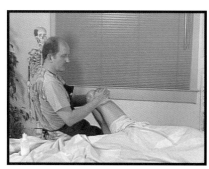

8. Hip Stretch

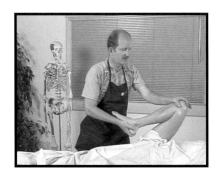

9. Hip Circumduction

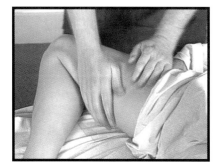

10. Figure 4 Adductor Stretch

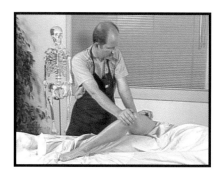

11. TFL Stroke

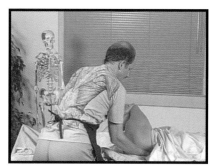

12. Piriformis

VIBRATION: Any sustained rhythm of movement in the body or body part induced by shaking, rocking or rolling. Because relaxed muscles tend to transmit the wave impetus more easily than tense muscles, vibration can be used to determine which parts of the body are harboring excessive tension. A rhythmical rocking of the whole body produces a profoundly sedative and comforting effect, reminiscent of the ocean or of being cradled in the womb. The calming effect of monotonous motion may allow a person to release chronically tense areas. Vibration is used after deep pressure or stretches to help the muscles release chronically held patterns of tension. The vibration offers momentary neurological confusion, allowing the muscles to re-pattern into a long lasting state of ease. Vigorous shaking or dis-synchronous movements may be of value in teaching a client to release a compulsive mental control of their musculature. Vibration is a very soothing and gentle way to begin or complete a massage.

STRETCHES: Any lengthening of a muscle group or connective tissue held at the point of maximum elongation for at least six seconds. All stretches should be done slowly and with care, being sensitive to the client's ability to release and relax with the stretch. Pay attention to nonverbal signs as well as verbal feedback, which indicate that the client may be experiencing discomfort, and adjust the stretch to insure their full relaxation. Stretches should never be done forcefully upon a contracted muscle because the muscle could go into a protective, reflex spasm, put an excessive strain on the tendons or possibly even tear. Stretches can be performed in stages allowing the muscle to release, rest and release further.

It is very important during a stretch to match the fullest extension with the client's exhalation. Verbal guidance through the stretch is often desirable. After a thorough stretch, the area should be gently vibrated or rocked to help re-pattern the muscle into a deeper degree of relaxation.

Benefits of stretching include increased flexibility, increased range of motion to joints, enhanced overall mobility, promotion of circulation by reducing muscular tension and heightening body awareness.

DEEP PRESSURE: Deep pressure is a highly relative term used to describe the maximum amount of pressure required to release tension from or strip toxins out of a muscle, while staying within the client's parameters of comfort. Deep pressure also releases adhesions between layers of fascia, giving greater mobility across joints and allowing positive postural changes. The mechanics of deep pressure work can be accomplished with fingertip, thumb, knuckle or elbow pressure applied steadily to specific muscle groups. All deep pressure work should be done slowly. It may be a stationary, steady pressure applied to a 'knotted' area, or a sliding pressure (generally along the grain of the muscle) or even applied in small circles around a specific point.

Deep pressure requires working right on the fine line of a clients ability to stay relaxed. The therapist must employ a great deal of sensitivity in this process. It is important that the client has complete trust in the therapist and knows that the therapist will adjust the pressure according to their verbal or even nonverbal responses. To ensure this always

begin lightly and move to deeper levels progressively, identifying areas of greater tenderness and verifying your rapport or ability to accurately gauge the client's comfort level. Make sure that your movements and words are in themselves calm and confident. Set up some kind of verbal feedback system to monitor specifically the preferred pressure.

Begin by clarifying the difference between a pressure that "hurts so good" versus the experience of pain or even fear of pain that causes resistance. It may be enough to simply ask for a signal if the pressure approaches "pain", or you may elect to use a numerical scale that reflects their comfort range of pressure. Be aware that the pressure required may vary in different areas of the body, just as much as it varies from person to person.

Occasionally a client may be incongruent between the verbal and nonverbal feedback they give you. In such cases they generally have the mistaken idea that "no pain = no gain". Re-educate them, explaining how muscle release cannot take place when the muscle is simultaneously bracing itself for pain! Continue only when you have their cooperation to stay in touch and give honest feedback.

Often times there can be an emotional release in conjunction with a physical release. We tend to store up memories of certain traumatic events in body parts associated with that trauma. If this occurs, do not back off from the work unless the client specifically requests it. Let your client know that it is OK to express what they are feeling and that it is part of a healing process. It is, however, not usually advisable to openly encourage emotional release, unless you have been properly trained in specific facilitation skills.

ENERGY CHANNELING: Energy channeling is the conscious and focused directing of the flow of life energy to enhance the healing another human being. It is as timeless as love itself and can be done whenever there is a pure heart focused on the well being of another. A perfect example of this is when a mother holds and comforts her infant child who is ill, and the child will become calmer and more comfortable. In massage, it can be incorporated gracefully by allowing your hands to linger in the area that intuitively draws you, and visualizing healing energy flowing through your hands into the client's body; balancing and aiding the body to heal itself. You may develop a refined sensitivity to the quality of energy moving throughout the body and augment your work by a focused intention to open energy blockages. This work can be surprisingly powerful and is best not attempted without permission or a request from your client. Always be certain you are properly grounded and clear in your own intent before and during this work. I have also found it helpful to ask for the guidance and protection of this person's higher self. The hands will often become warm during energy channeling; this is simply the focused flow of energy moving within the healing space you've created. The laying on of hands is noted in the bible and in the spiritual practices of many peoples, and as with all things, is a bit of a mystery to us. Yet, it is an undeniable gift for those that wish to recognize and embrace it without fear.

Torso Stroke Sequence – Male Client

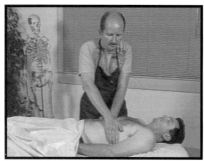

1. Rocking Rib Cage

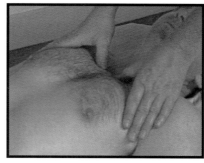

2. Lymphatic Release

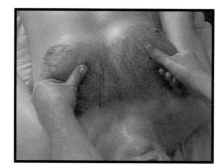

3. Pectoralis Major

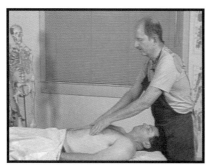

4. Rib Cage

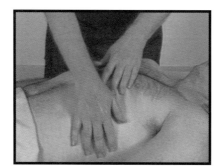

5. Raking Intercostals

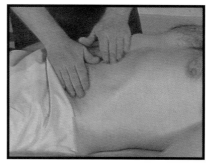

6. Colon Chase

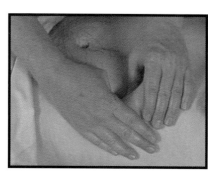

7. Diaphragm Release

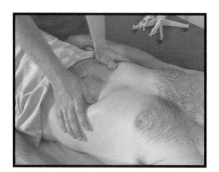

8. Diamond

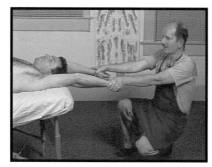

9. Arm Overhead Stretch

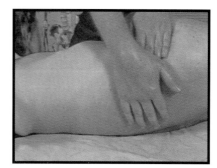

10. Side Lift

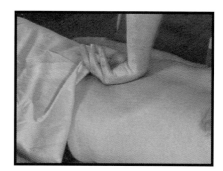

11. Corkscrew

Cautions and Contraindications of Massage

Cautions

1. Pain – Sometimes pain must be induced to secure results, such as in stretching adhesions and in the treatment of fibrositis in muscles or subcutaneous tissue, but generally there is no pain or discomfort in massage. Clients should be educated about the difference between pain being released and pain being inflicted.

2. Alcohol – do not ingest alcohol within 24 hours of a massage;

3. Diabetes – go lightly on legs and feet, clients may have nerve and circulatory problems in advanced cases of diabetes.

4. Certain prescription drugs – be cautious if the client is taking any of the following:

5.
   Pain Medication - clients can't give adequate feedback
   Heart Medication - get doctors permission for massage
   Blood Pressure Medication - check if blood pressure is controlled
   Corticosteroids - increased risk of osteoporosis
   BloodThinners - client may be taking these because of risk of blood clots.

Inflammation

The suffix "-itis" means inflammation. Inflammation is characterized by four signs: Redness, Swelling, Heat, and Pain.

Massage is contraindicated where there is inflammation as it may further inflame an area. The exception to this is with trigger point and counterstrain work when properly performed.

Contraindications

1. A swelling that might be a malignancy (controversial).

2. Skin infections or ulcerations.

3. Inflammation – whether local or deep.

4. Phlebitis, thrombosis or other vascular diseases.

5. Lymphangitis.

6. Acute fever.

7. Acute osteomyelitis, tubercular joints or any infectious bone or joint disease.

8. Where there is a tendency to hemorrhage – varicosities, peptic ulcers, menstruating uterus, hemophilia, and aneurisms.

9. Hypertension (High Blood Pressure) – Massage temporarily raises blood pressure before lowering it. Do not do vigorous massage on someone with hypertension.

10. Intermittent Claudication – symptoms are pain in the legs that gets worse upon exertion.

11. Pregnant uterus – generally.

12. Any conditions where there is impairment of nerve sensation, so that you may not get adequate feedback.

Disclaimer

Judiciously used, even in many of these conditions massage may greatly help the healing process. This list may not be complete so use your common sense. If in doubt about any conditions have your client get permission from their doctor for massage. The author of this book and Abundant Health Resources, Inc. dba as Hands On Healing, assume no liability for problems caused by the use or misuse of techniques discussed in this workbook and DVD.

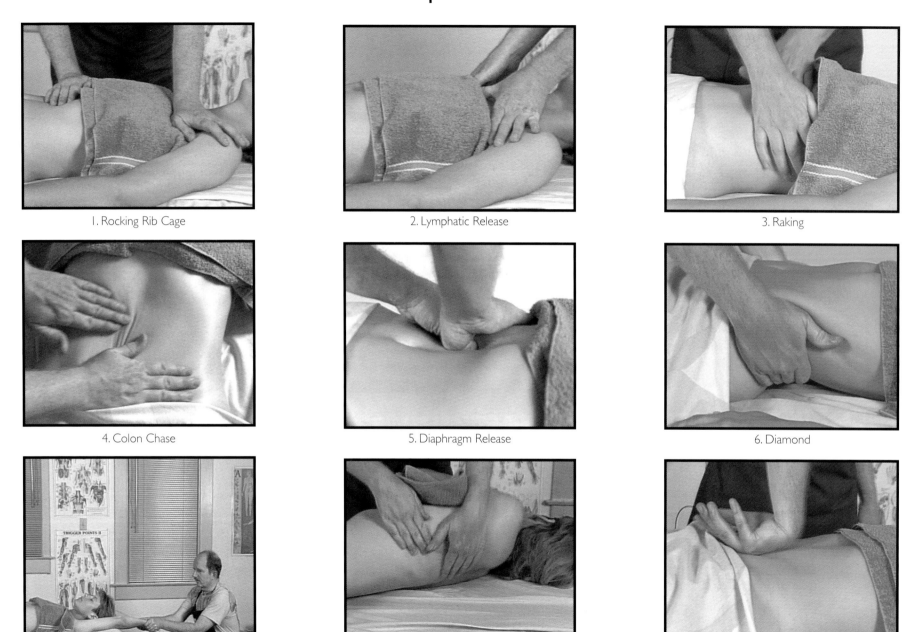

1. Rocking Rib Cage

2. Lymphatic Release

3. Raking

4. Colon Chase

5. Diaphragm Release

6. Diamond

7. Arm Overhead Stretch

8. Side Lift

9. Corkscrew

Long Stroke

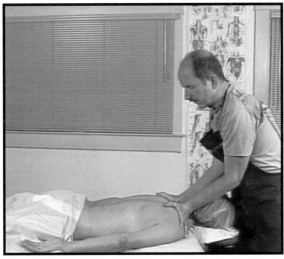

1. Heel press over the top of the shoulders.

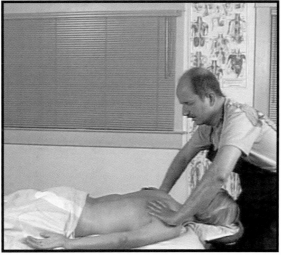

2. Pivot at the deltoids

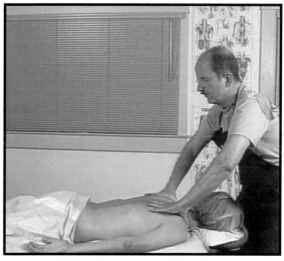

3. Thumbs across top of shoulders

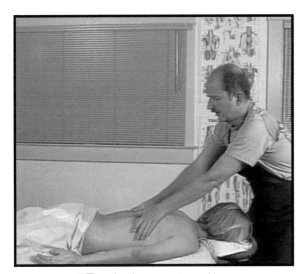

4. Thumbs down erector spinae

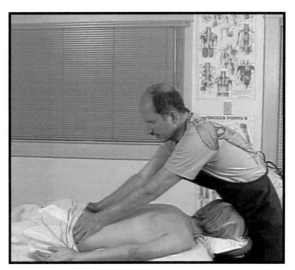

5. Heel press over sacrum

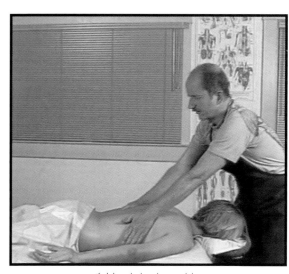

6. Hands back up sides

Arm Stroke Sequence

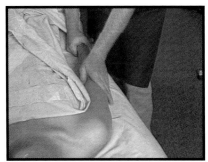
1. Long Stroke

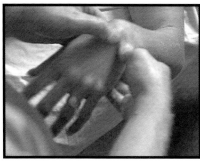
2. Wrist Articulation

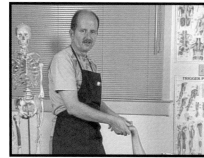
3. Metacarpal Grooves

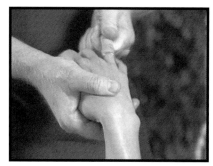
4. Articulate Fingers

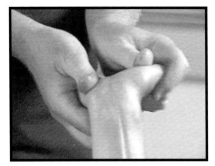
5. Palm Stretch

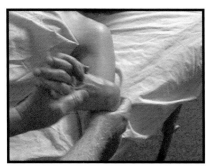
6. Wrist Circumduction

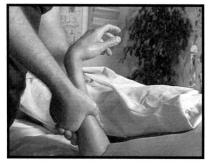
7. Ghost Hand

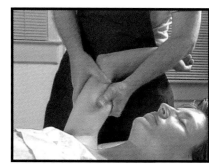
8. Arm Cradle

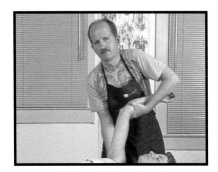
9. Deltoid, Rhomboids

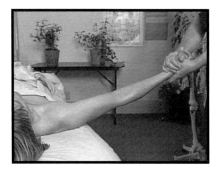
10. Shake Arm to Side

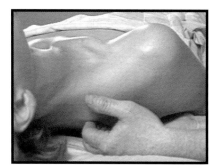
11. Bridging into Scapula

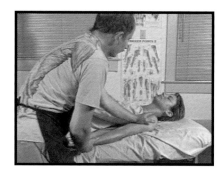
12. Arm Stretch

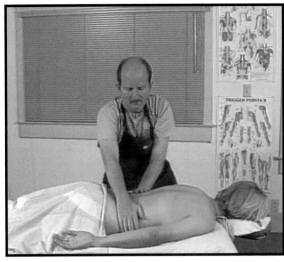
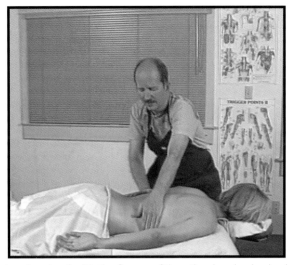
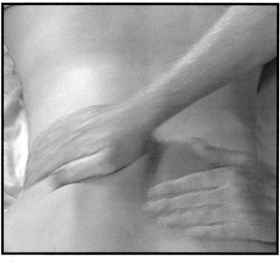

Press with the heel of one hand and pull with the fingers of the other hand going back and forth across the back.
Work from the iliac crest to the axilla, wrapping around the sides of the body. Allow your hips to move for better body mechanics.

Sacrum Heel Press

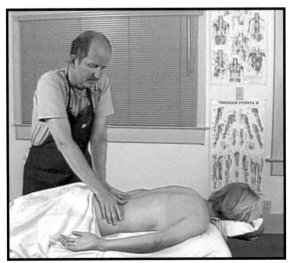
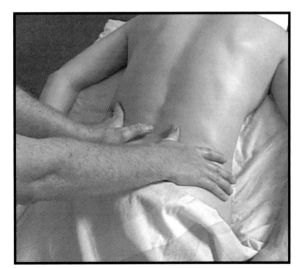
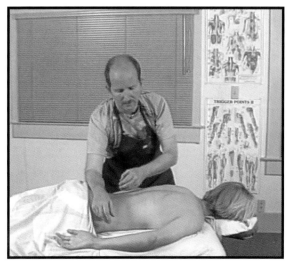

Press inferiorly on the sacrum with the heels of both hands, then separate your hands, gliding over the iliac crest.
An alternate technique is to press inferiorly on the sacrum with your forearm.

Neck Stroke Sequence

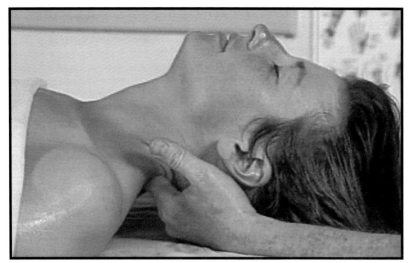

1. Lift and Pull

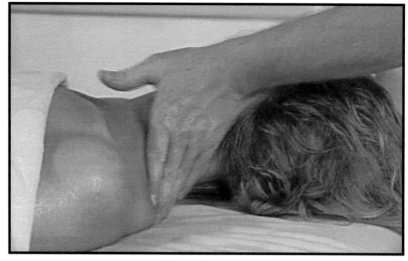

2. Trapezius Stroke

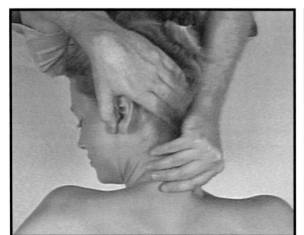

3. Levator Scapulae and Supraspinatus

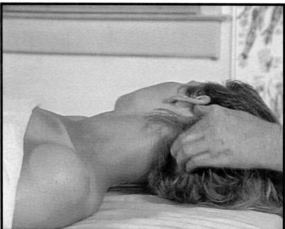

4. Occiput Circles

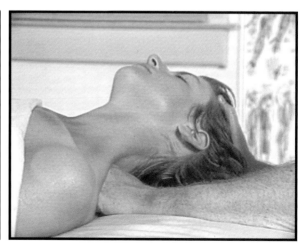

5. Lateral Flexion

Rolling Pin

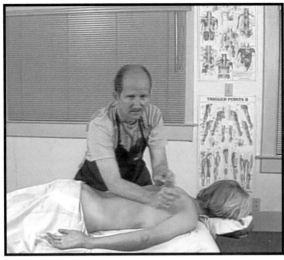
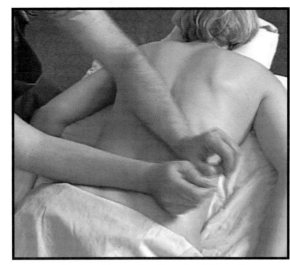
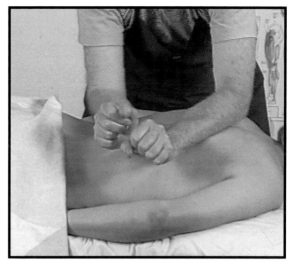

Use forearms to supply wide area pressure over back and buttocks. Care should be taken not to apply pressure directly over the spine.

Ironing

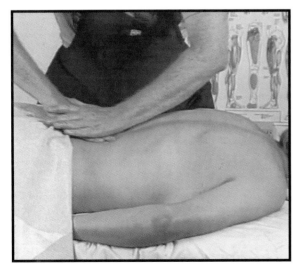
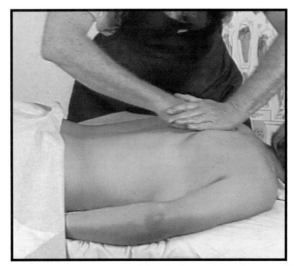
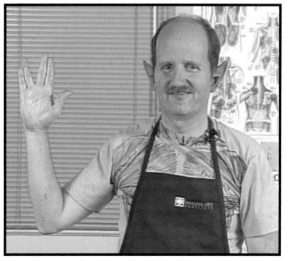

Spread fingers of bottom hand apart so that index and middle fingers are on one side of spine and ring finger and little finger are on the other side. Press the heel of your top hand onto the fingers of the bottom hand then glide up and down the spine, keeping the pressure on either side of the spine. Your bottom hand stays relaxed, the pressure is applied through the heel of the top hand.

Face Stroke Sequence

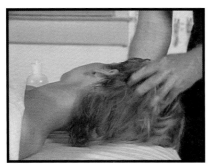
1. Scalp Shampoo

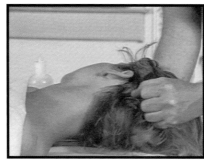
2. Hair Pull Circles

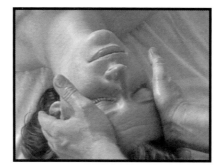
3. Forehead Heel Press

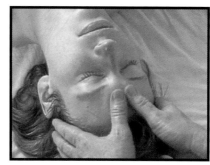
4. Brow Clearing with Thumbs

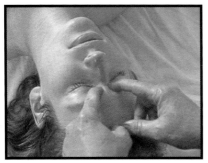
5. Supraorbital Ridge

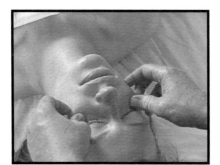
6. Infraorbital Ridge

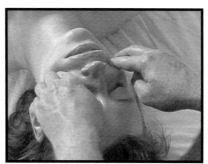
7. Cheekbone Plough

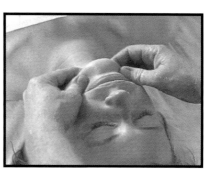
8. Define Maxilla and Mandible

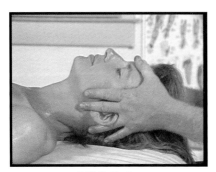
9. TMJ Circles

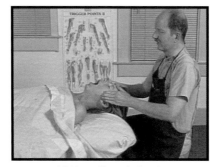
10. Yawn Stretch Stroke

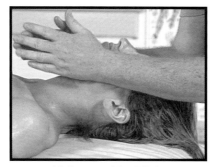
11. Forearm Hand Slide

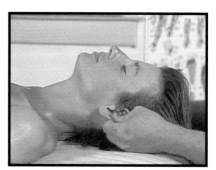
12. Ear Massage

Scapula Work

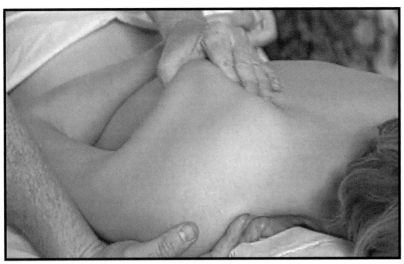

1. With client's forearm behind their back knead around the medial and axillary borders of the scapula.

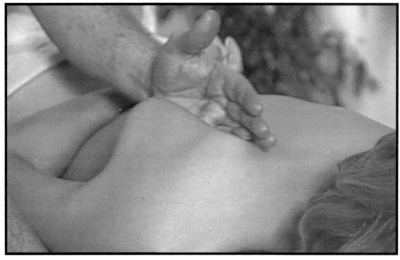

2. Do a sawing motion with the lateral side of your hand under the medial border of the scapula.

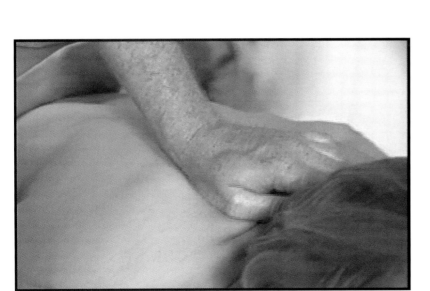

3. Work the rhomboids from the medial border of the scapula toward the spine with the heel of your hand.

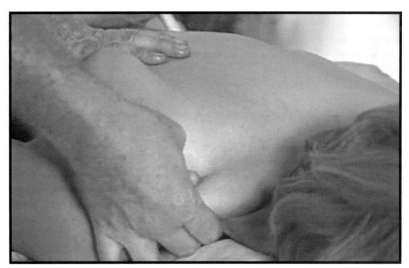

4. Knead the upper trapezius and supraspinatus with your outside hand.

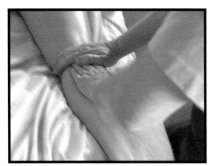

1. Long Stroke

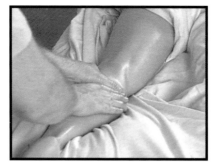

2. V Stroke

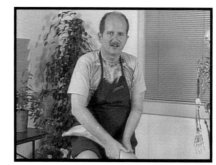

3. Runners Delight

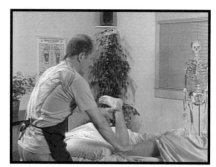

4. Windshield Wiper

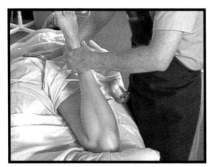

5. Quadriceps Stretch

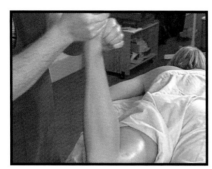

6. Leg Lift and Wobble

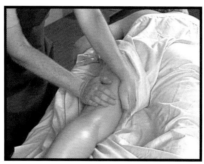

7. Kneading Hamstrings

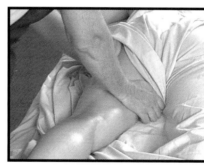

8. Fulling Hamstrings

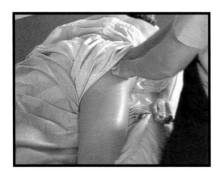

9. Knuckle Rub

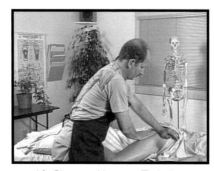

10. Glutes – Alternate Technique

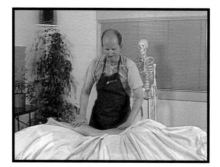

11. Rocking and Vibration

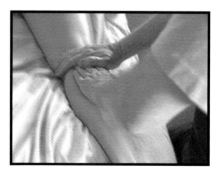

12. Long Stroke

Pectoralis Stretch Stroke

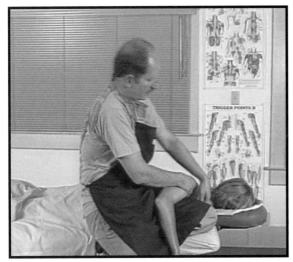

Have client's arm draped across your knee.

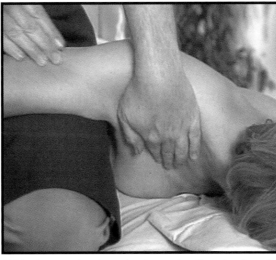

With alternate hands stroke the pectoralis major from its origin on the sternum to its insertion on the humerus.

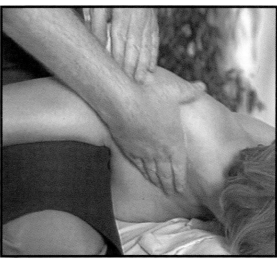

Be sure to stay inferior to the clavicle with your strokes.

Petrissage Deltoid, Triceps

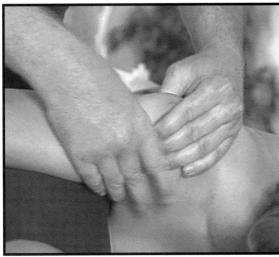

In this same position you can petrissage the deltoid and the triceps.

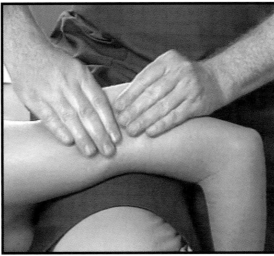

Torquing

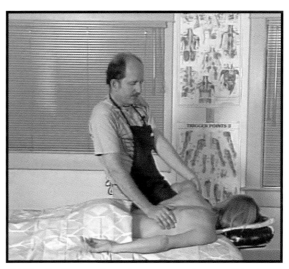

With client's arm draped across your knee, pull back on the shoulder with one hand while gliding up the opposite side of the spine with the other hand.

Back Stroke Sequence

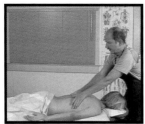
1. Long Stroke

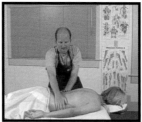
2. Side to Side

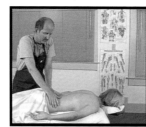
3. Sacrum Heel Press

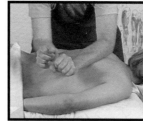
4. Rolling Pin

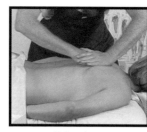
5. Ironing

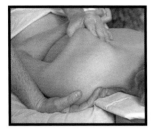
6. Scapula - Kneading

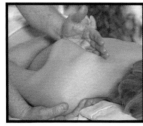
7. Scapula - Sawing

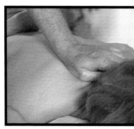
8. Rhomboids

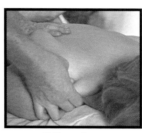
9. Kneading Upper Trapezius

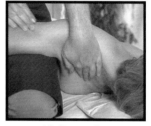
10. Pectoralis Stretch Stroke

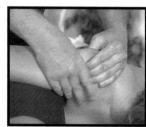
11. Petrissage Deltoids

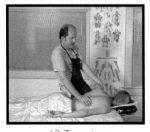
12. Torquing

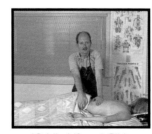
13. Hip Lift and Glide

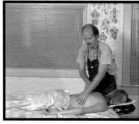
14. Raking

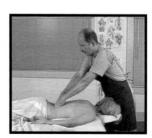
15. Knuckles down Erector Spinae

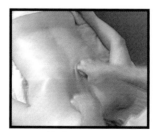
16. Scrubbing

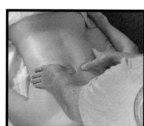
17. Pressure Points

Strokes 6 - 14 should be repeated on the other side of the back.

Hip Lift and Glide

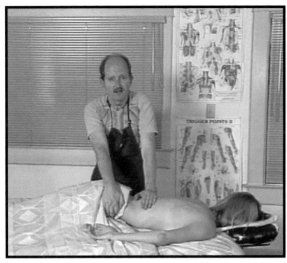 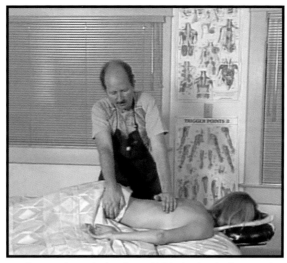 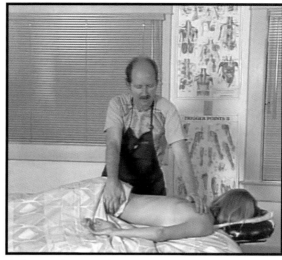

Using your body weight, gently lift the ASIS with your fingers through the drape. With the heel of your other hand glide up the side of the spine opposite you.

Raking

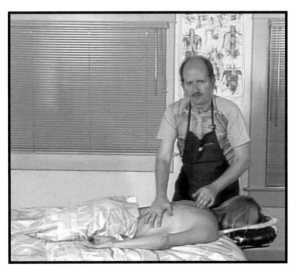 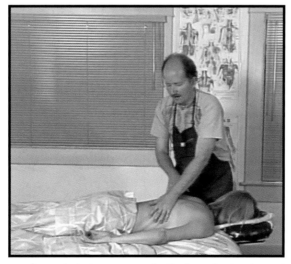 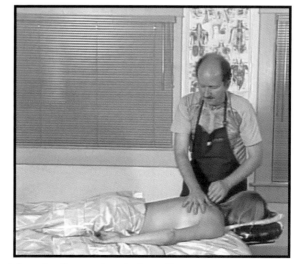

Standing by your client's shoulder, glide your fingers in between your client's ribs, going hand over hand from the iliac crest up to the axilla.

EXTRA STROKES
Side Lift – Variation

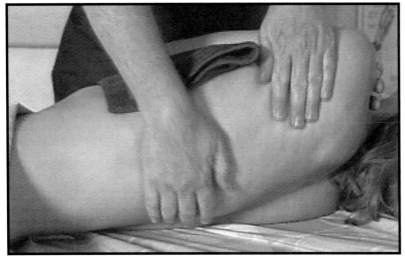 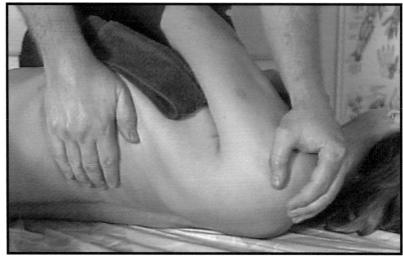

Do a side lift working hand over hand, lifting the client with a hand over hand motion. Then gently press shoulder down with one hand while lifting the client's side with the other hand.

Neck Stretch

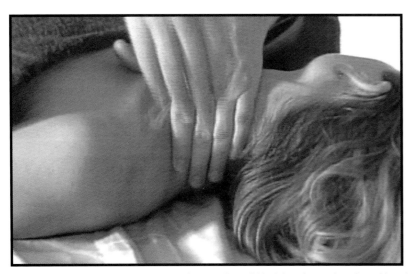 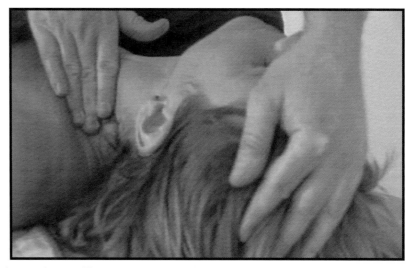

Have your client's head turned toward you. Work hand over hand stroking side of client's neck opposite you. Then rotate your client's head away from you while stroking back toward you. Do not stroke over the front of the neck.

Knuckles Down Erector Spinae

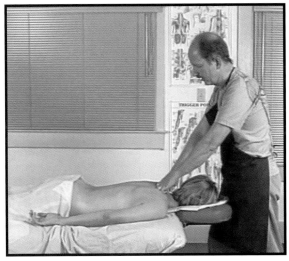
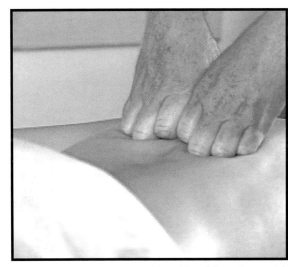
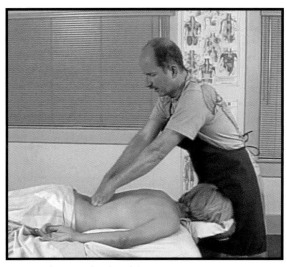

With your proximal interphalangeal joints in a row glide down either side of the spine applying pressure using your bodyweight.
Do not press directly on the spinous processes of the vertebrae.

Scrubbing

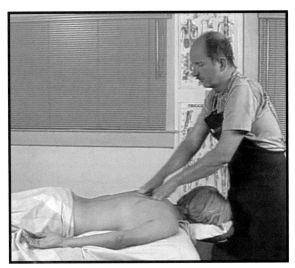
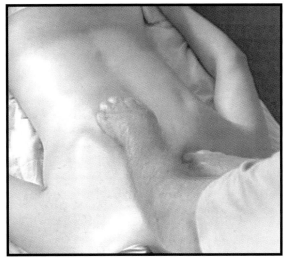
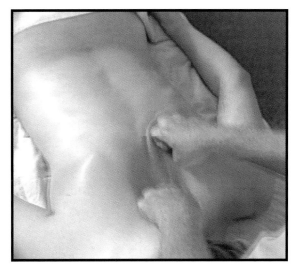

Using a push pull motion with your knuckles work on either side of the spine applying friction.

FINISHING STROKES
Rocking Feet

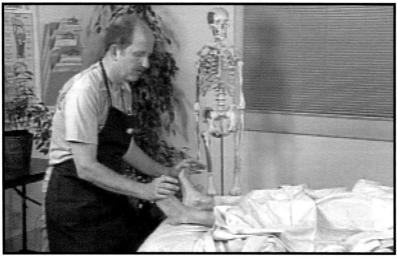 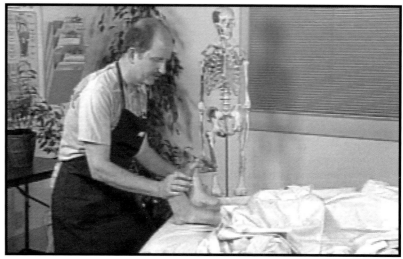

With the heels of your hands press and release the balls of your client's feet so that your client's whole body rocks.
Find the rhythm that works best for your client's body.

Rocking Umbilicus

Thumbs over Eyes

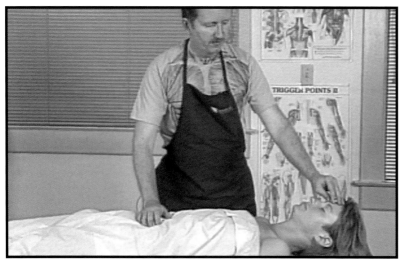 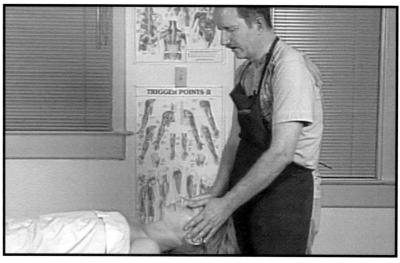

Place right hand on umbilicus and left hand on brow.
Gently rock umbilicus.

Place your thumbs gently over your client's closed eyes.

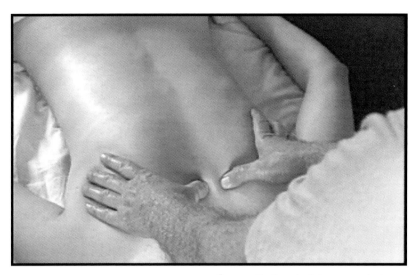 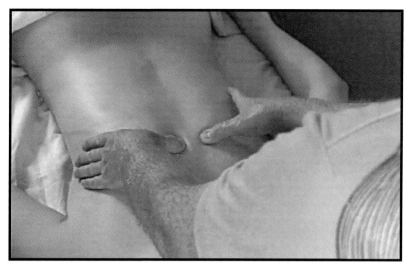

Press with thumbs into spaces between transverse processes on either side of your client's spine.
You can work down the spine, over the notches in the sacrum, and around the iliac crest, holding each point for several seconds

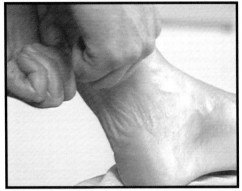

1. Working into arch with fingers

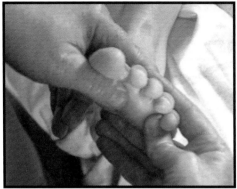

2. Thumbands into metatarsal space

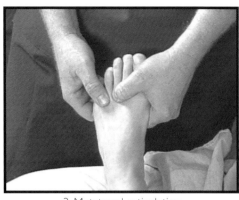

3. Metatarsal articulation

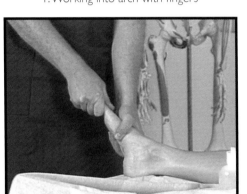

4. Toe articulation and pull

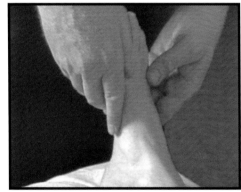

5. Tendon Grooves on dorsal surface

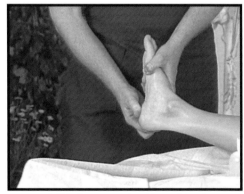

6. Friction around ankle and heel

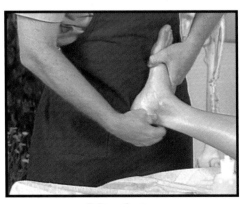

7. Dorsiflexion

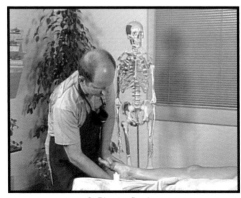

8. Plantarflexion

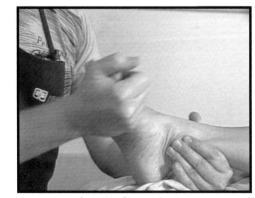

9. Ankle Circumduction

This is only one of many ways to massage the feet.

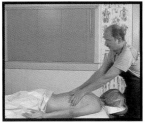

1. Long Stroke

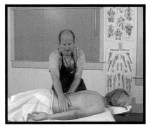

2. Side to Side

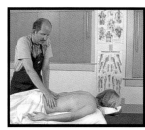

3. Sacrum Heel Press

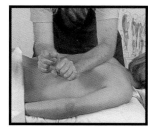

4. Rolling Pin

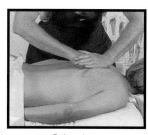

5. Ironing

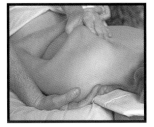

6. Scapula - Kneading

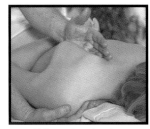

7. Scapula - Sawing

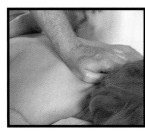

8. Rhomboids

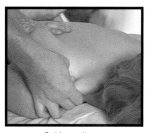

9. Kneading
Upper Trapezius

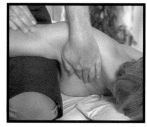

10. Pectoralis
Stretch Stroke

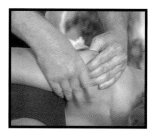

11. Petrissage Deltoids

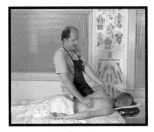

12. Torquing

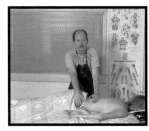

13. Hip Lift and Glide

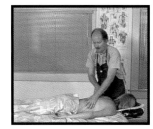

14. Raking

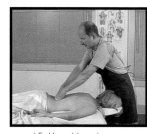

15. Knuckles down
Erector Spinae

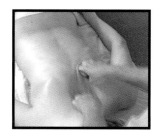

16. Scrubbing

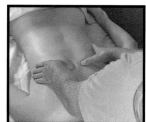

17. Pressure Points

Strokes 6-14 should be repeated on the other side.
This is only one of many ways to massage the back.

Dorsiflexion

Plantarflexion

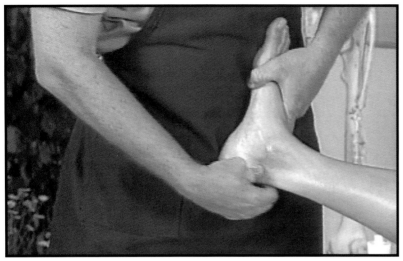

Dorsiflex ankle while working around achilles tendon.

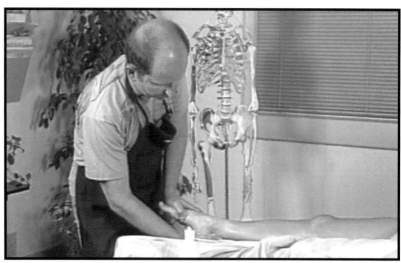

Plantarflex ankle.

Ankle Circumduction

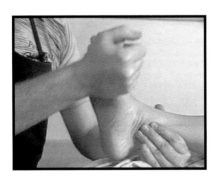 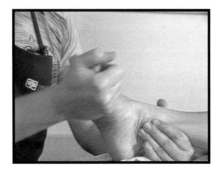 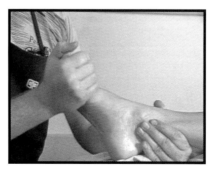 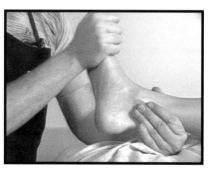

Place one hand proximal to the ankle joint and one hand around the ball of the foot. Do full slow circumduction of the ankle joint.

Long Stroke

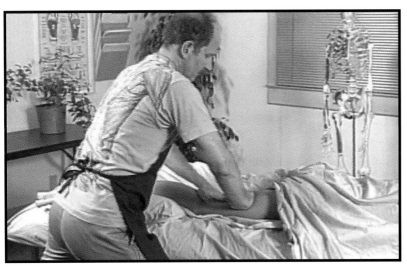
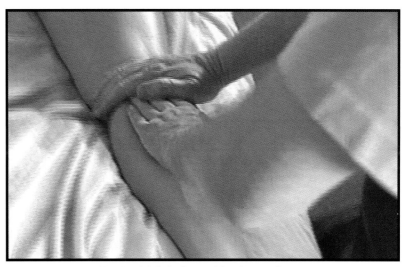

Both hands effleurage from achilles tendon toward ischium, firm pressure up leg and light pressure down. Leading hand leads with little finger side of hand. Go lighter over popliteal area and over varicose veins. Pressure is applied only when working in a proximal direction (toward the heart). Go lighter when coming back down the leg.

V Stroke

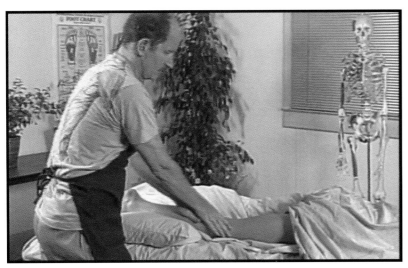
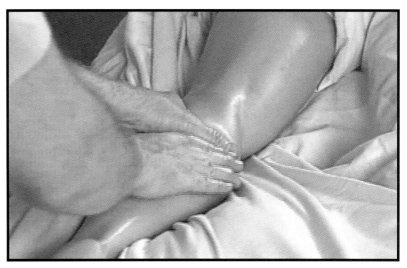

A long stroke using the "V" between thumb and fingers to provide more specific pressure.
Pressure is applied only when working in a proximal direction (toward the heart). Go lighter when coming back down the leg.

Tendon Grooves

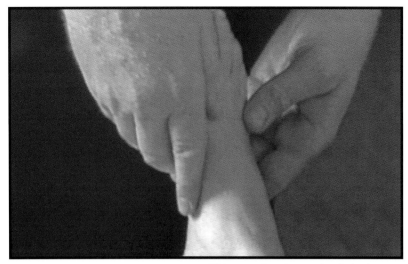 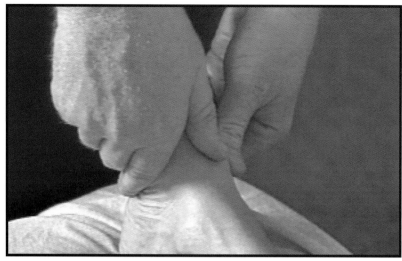

Slide your thumbs proximally in the grooves between the tendons on the dorsal surface of the foot.

Friction Around Ankle and Heel

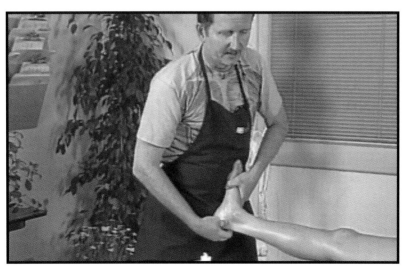 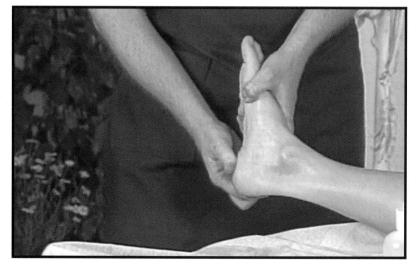

Apply friction with your thumbs all around the ankle joint and heel.

Runner's Delight

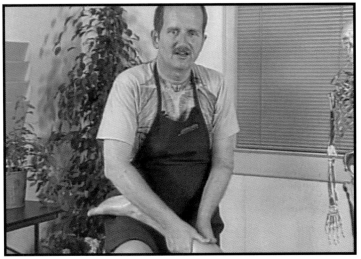
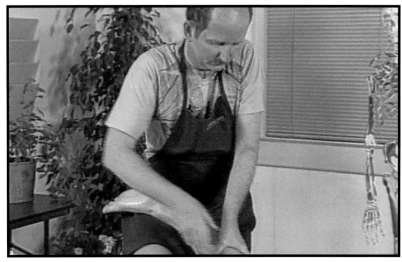

Starting from achilles tendon, work circular thumbs through gastrocnemius, thumb bands across top of calf. Return with glide lifting back of calf, defining soleus down to achilles tendon attachment at ankle.

Windshield Wiper

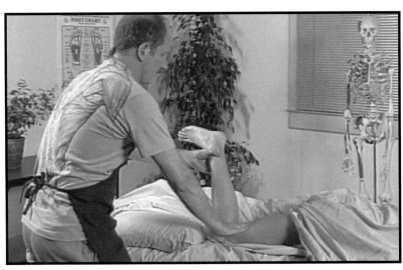
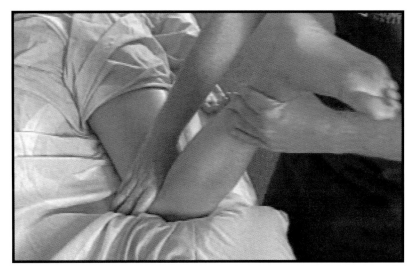

With client's knee flexed, pull leg side to side while working popliteal space with the web between thumb and index finger of other hand.

Metatarsal Articulation

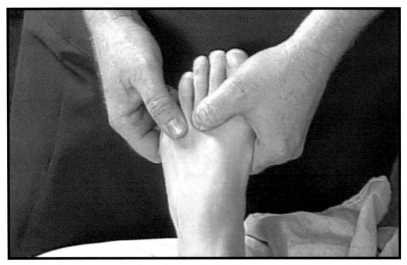
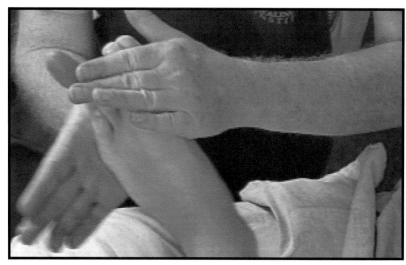

Move adjacent metatarsals against each other in an up and down motion. This can be done with individual metatarsals, or you can articulate all the metatarsals at the same time by cupping your hands around either side of the foot then squeezing the foot and moving your hands back and forth vigorously.

Toe Articulation and Pull

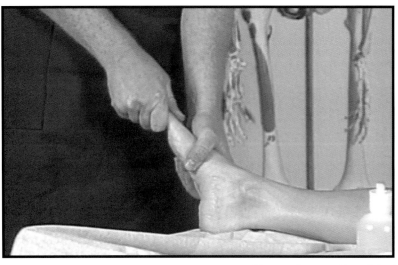
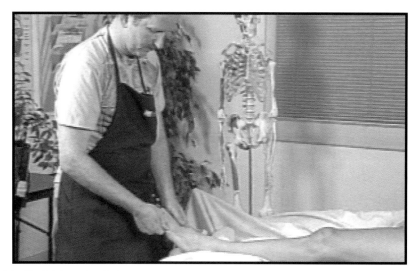

Massage toes working all the joints, then articulate the joints and pull the toes.

Quad Stretch

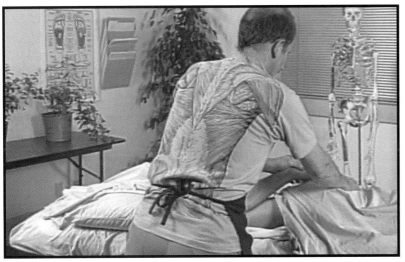

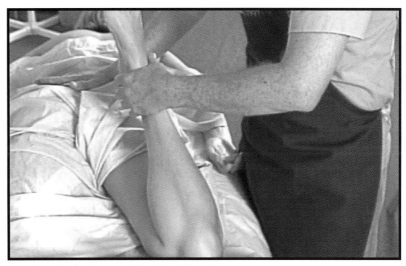

Bring client's heel toward buttocks, while pressing inferiorly on sacrum. Stretch slowly especially with older clients.
For an extra stretch place your knee on the table and rest client's thigh over your knee.

Leg Lift and Wobble

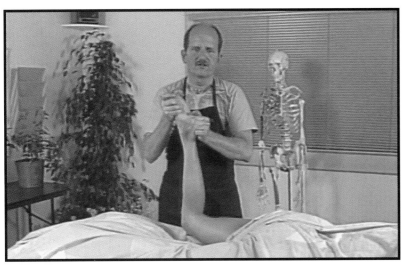

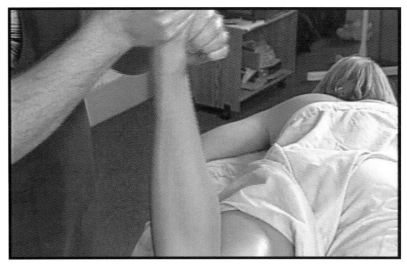

Hold client's foot at heel and ball of foot. Lift foot so that knee is off the table then gently shake entire leg.

Working into Arch with Fingers

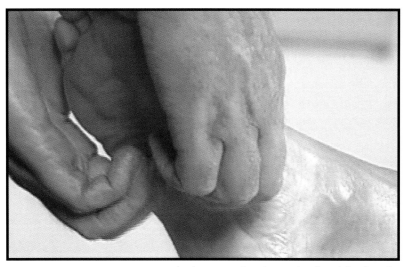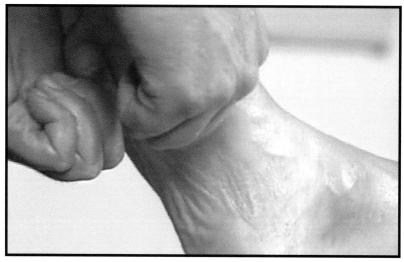

Anchor your thumbs on the dorsal (top) surface of the foot, then stroke the plantar (bottom) surface of the foot
with your fingers pulling toward you. Do not let the thumbs slide as that can be painful.

Thumb Bands into Metatarsal Space

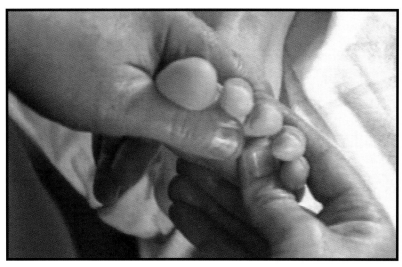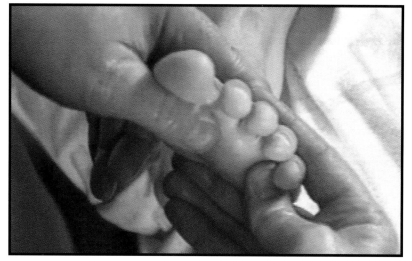

Place your thumbs next to each other by the third metatarsal head, then slide them apart with pressure to the metatarsal heads.

Kneading Hamstrings

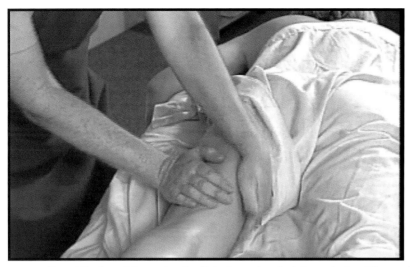 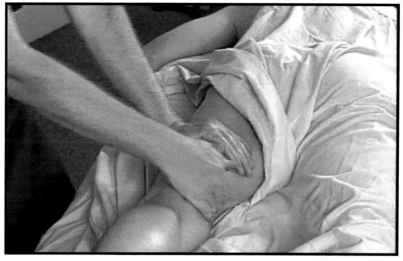

Knead the hamstrings using the flat of your hands doing wringing, lifting and squeezing. Press with the heel of one hand while pulling with the fingers of the other hand.

Fulling Hamstrings

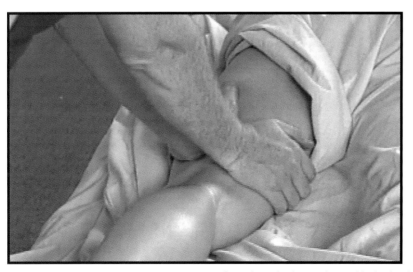 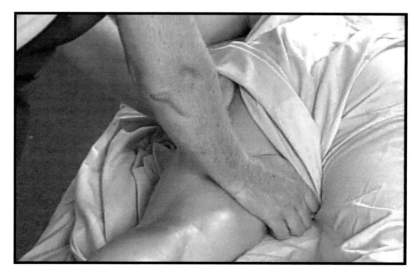

Press into the hamstrings with the heels of your hands and move them in opposite directions.

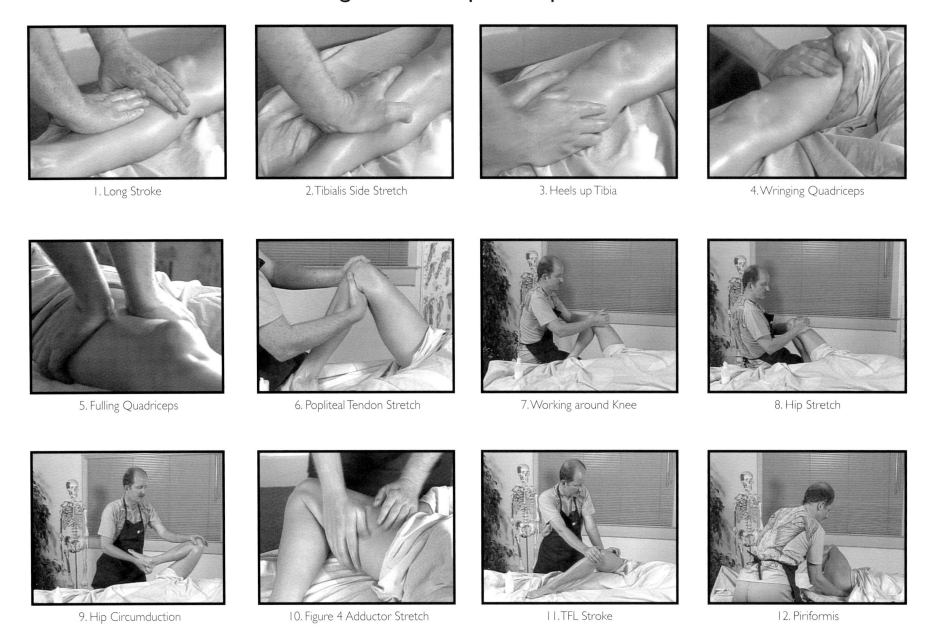

1. Long Stroke

2. Tibialis Side Stretch

3. Heels up Tibia

4. Wringing Quadriceps

5. Fulling Quadriceps

6. Popliteal Tendon Stretch

7. Working around Knee

8. Hip Stretch

9. Hip Circumduction

10. Figure 4 Adductor Stretch

11. TFL Stroke

12. Piriformis

This is only one of many ways to massage the front of the legs.

Knuckle Rub

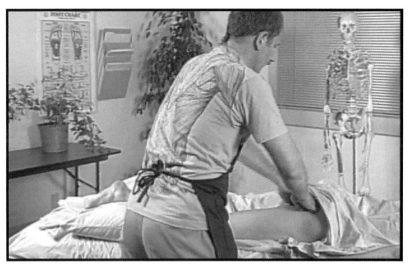

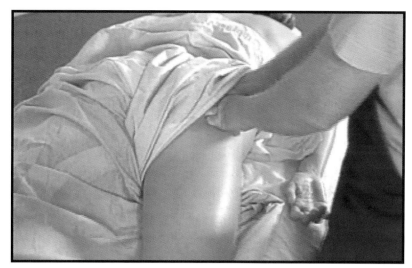

Interlock thumbs and move knuckles together in figure eight pattern over gluteal area.

Glutes – Alternate Technique

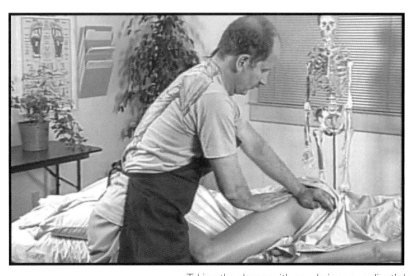

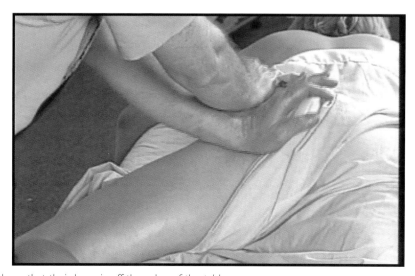

Taking the drape with you, bring your client's leg out to the side so that their knee is off the edge of the table.
Brace against their knee with your leg and work with the heels of your hands superiorly and laterally in the arc between the greater trochanter and the sacrum and iliac crest.

Tensor Fascia Lata Stroke

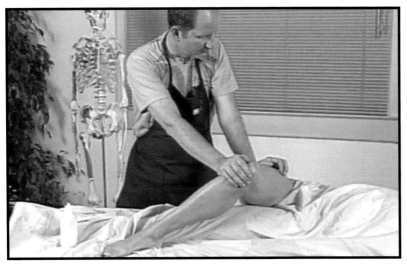
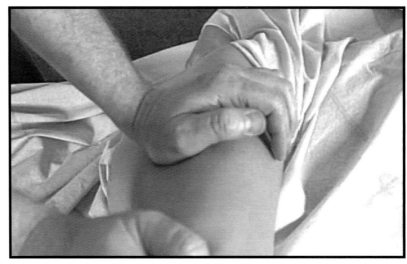

Knee flexed, position foot crossed over opposite leg. Heel of outside hand strokes slowly and firmly down lateral side of leg, inside hand supports client's knee or stretches, depending on relative tightness of TFL.

Piriformis

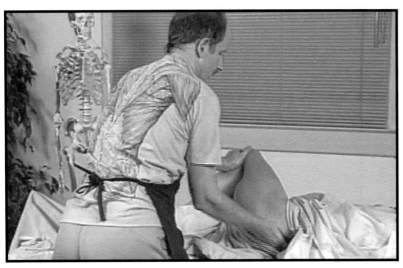
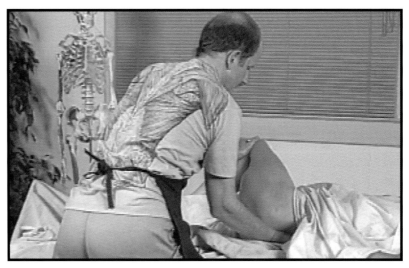

With your client in same position as for TFL stroke work with the heel of your hand going from the greater trochanter to the sacrum. Press your client's knee away from you to maximize the stretch.

Rocking and Vibration

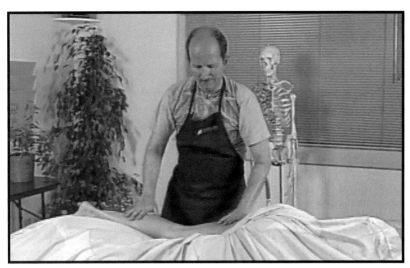

Place hands on client's leg and rock gently.

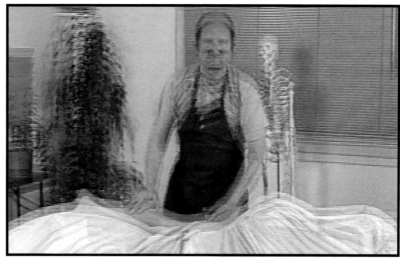

Do not rock vigorously!

Hip Circumduction

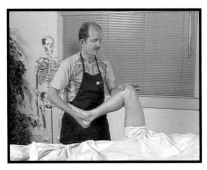 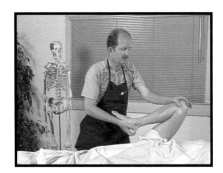 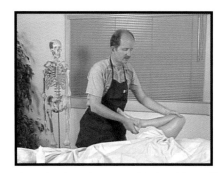 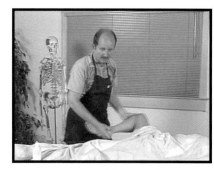

Full slow circumduction of hip keeping ankle on an imaginary line running inferior from hip and moving knee in an arc. Begin with small circular movements to define comfort range. Be careful to support leg completely so that it won't hyperextend at knee. Draping should be carefully maintained to ensure client's privacy.

Figure 4 Adductor Stretch Stroke

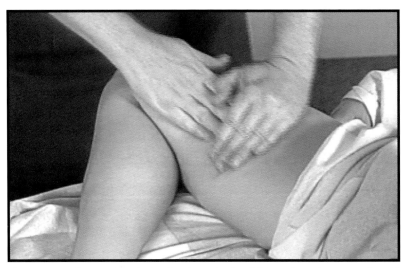 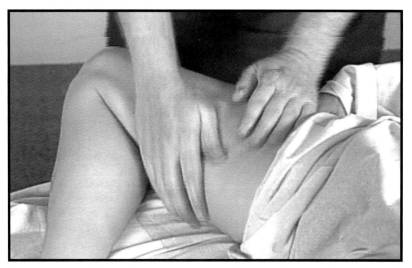

Place client's foot against their other knee, let leg fall laterally as far as comfortable, then push gently down on knee while stroking up adductors with palm or forearm. Discretion and sensitivity should be used as the adductor attachments are often very tense.

Leg Strokes Prone Sequence

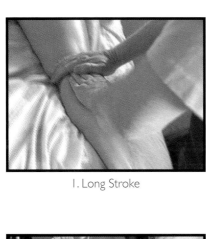

1. Long Stroke

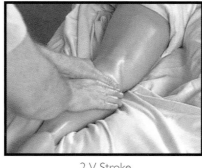

2. V Stroke

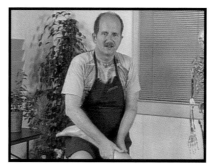

3. Runner's Delight

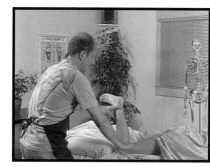

4. Windshield Wiper

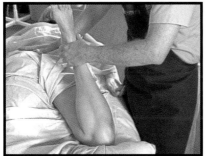

5. Quadriceps Stretch

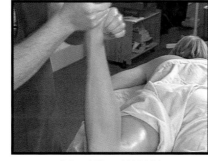

6. Leg Lift and Wobble

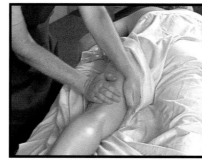

7. Kneading Hamstrings

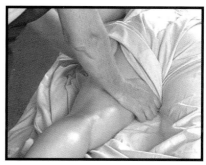

8. Fulling Hamstrings

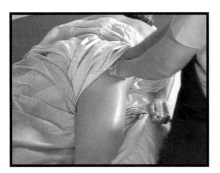

9. Knuckle Rub

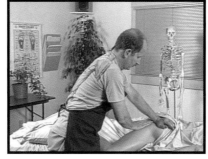

10. Glutes – Alternate Technique

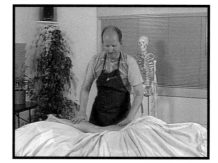

11. Rocking and Vibration

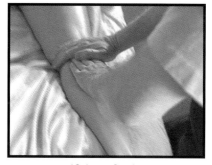

12. Long Stroke

This is only one of many ways to massage the back of the legs.

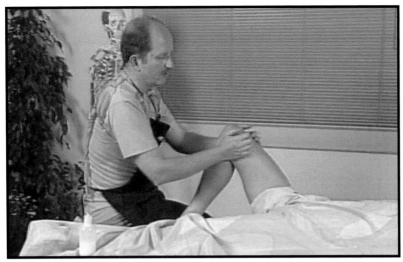 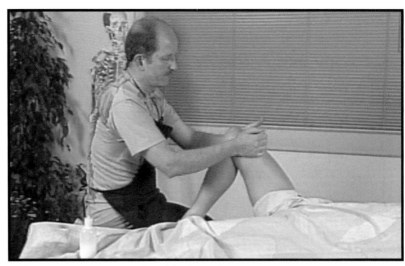

Work with a circular motion around both sides of knee. For clients with hairy knees use a back and forth motion.

Hip Stretch

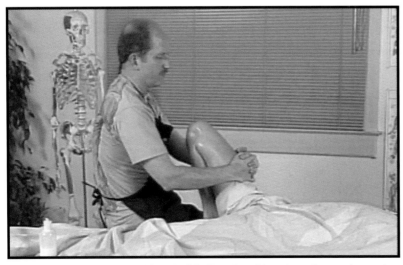 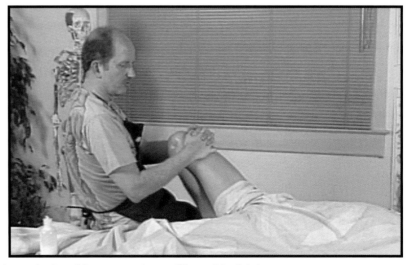

Knee in fully flexed position, sit on foot and wrap hands just above the knee; slowly pull knee towards you, lifting pelvis slightly.

Scalp Shampoo

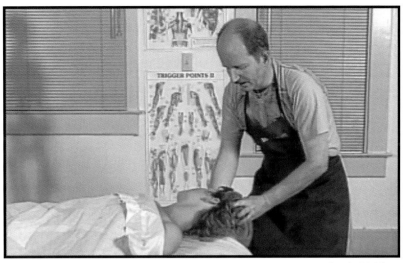

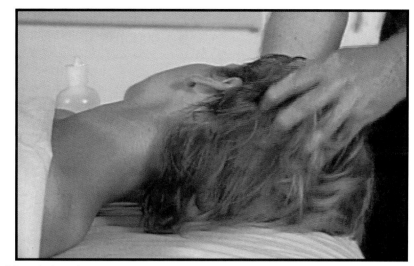

Semi-rigid fingertip scrubbing of the whole scalp.

Hair Pull Circles

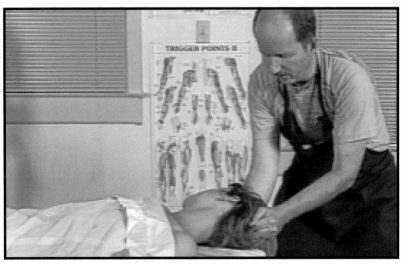

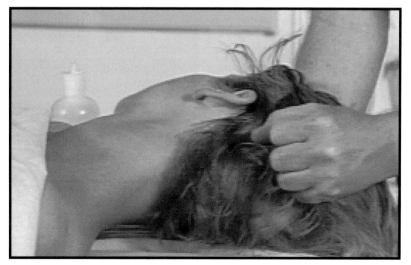

Clasp a handful of hair at root and hold securely. Pressing your closed fist against the scalp, make small circles.

Fulling Quadriceps

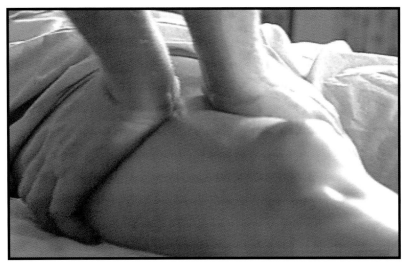 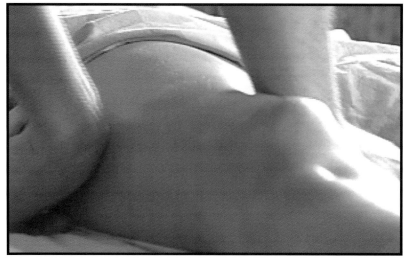

Press on the quadriceps with the heels of your hands moving apart from each other.

Popliteal Tendon Stretch

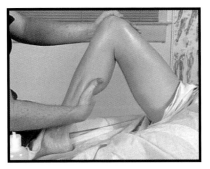 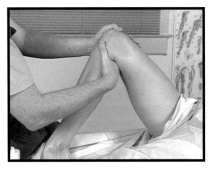 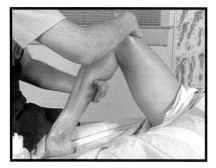 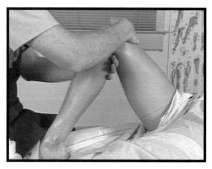

Client's knee flexed to 90 degrees, sole of client's foot on table, hands alternately glide up calf into popliteal space and stretch each tendon outwards, other hand stabilizes knee. Stroke all the way from the achilles tendon to the hamstring tendons. One hand pulls the tendons medially then the other hand pulls the tendons laterally.

Forehead Heel Press

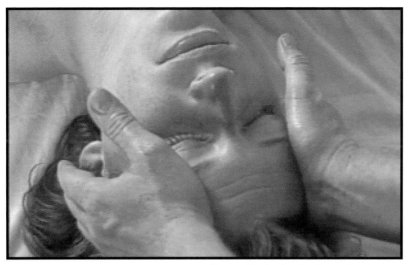 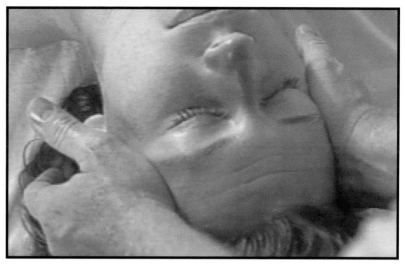

Press with the heels of your hands across the forehead, starting at the middle and moving outward.

Brow Clearing with Thumbs

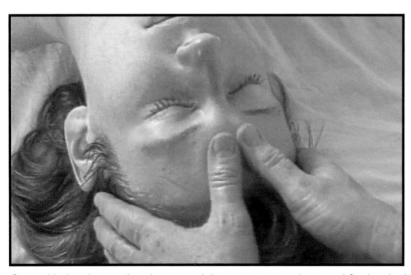 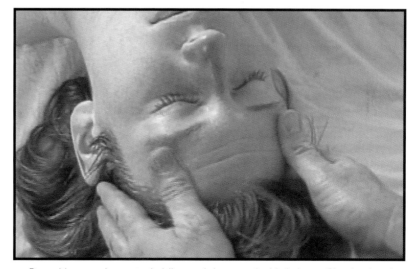

Start with thumbs together, then spread them apart across brow and forehead using medium pressure. Reposition, moving up to hairline and down again. Variation – Circular thumbs.

Heels Up Tibia

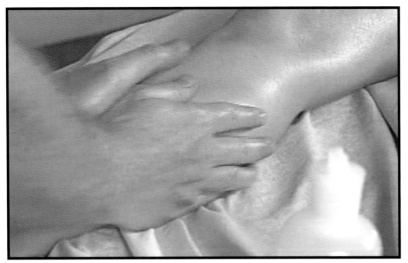
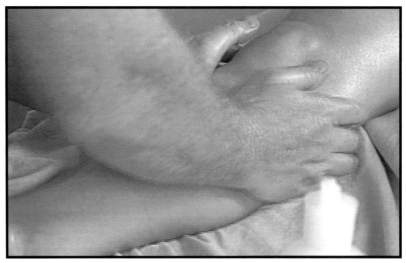

Move heels of hands superiorly while pressing hands towards each other on both sides of tibia.

Wringing Quadriceps

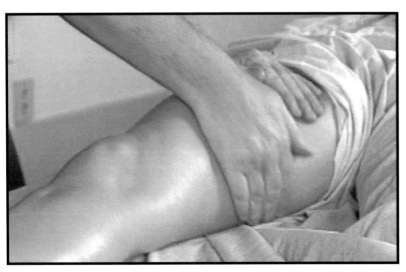
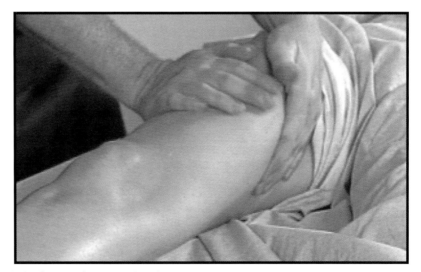

Press with the heel of one hand while pulling with the fingers of the other hand.

Supraorbital Ridge

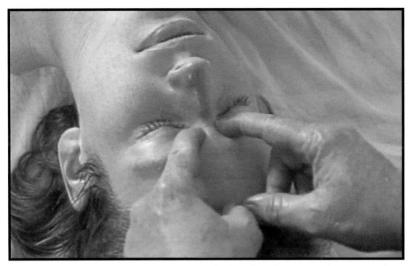 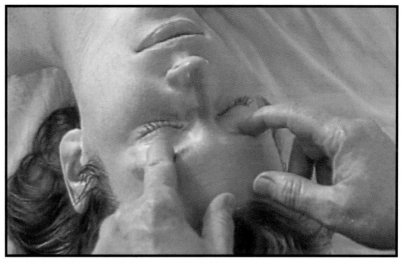

Ascertain the client is not wearing contact lenses. Go point by point with fingertips around the supraorbital ridge.
Pressure is applied superiorly into the arch of the bone. Do not put pressure on eye.

Infraorbital Ridge

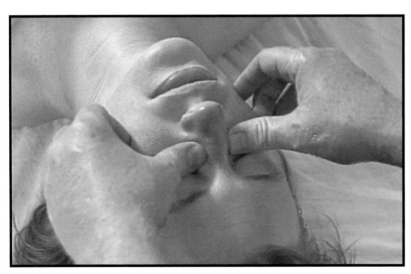 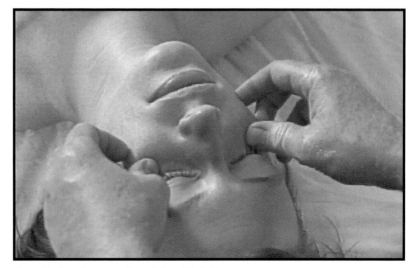

Ascertain the client is not wearing contact lenses. Go point by point with thumbs around the infraorbital ridge.
Pressure is applied inferiorly into the arch of the bone. Do not put pressure on eye or drag thumbs.

Long Stroke

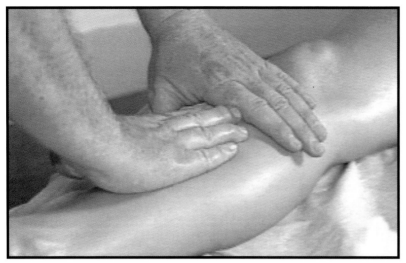 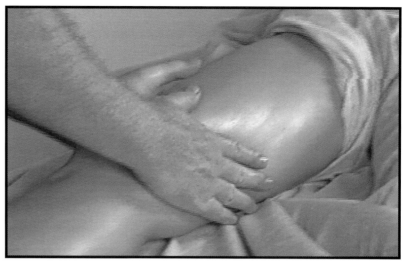

Both hands firm effleurage from ankle to top of leg, fulling just below groin area, return with light effleurage down back of leg.
Leading hand leads with little finger side of hand.

Tibialis Side Stretch

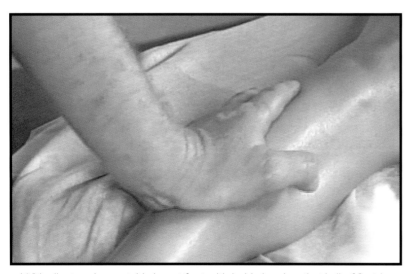 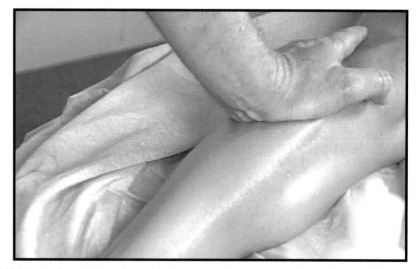

With client supine on table invert foot with inside hand so that ball of foot is pressing on table. With heel of outside hand, or with forearm, stroke up peroneal muscles and tibialis anterior on lateral side of tibia, pressing these muscles medially into the bone.

Cheekbone Plough

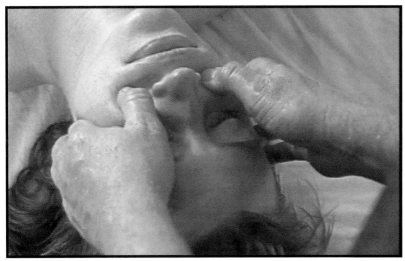

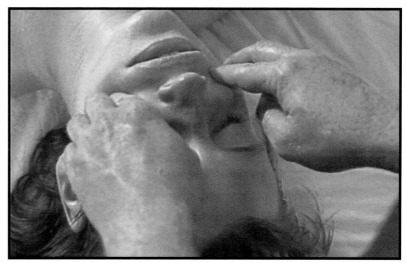

Use fingertips or thumbs to stoke inferior to zygomatic arch moving from nose to ear.

Define Maxilla

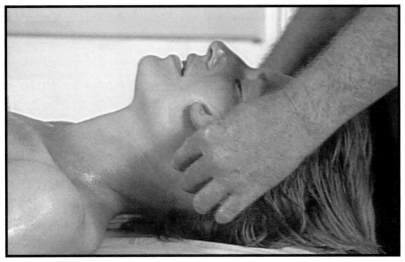

Define the upper jaw with your thumbs moving from the midline outward.

Define Mandible

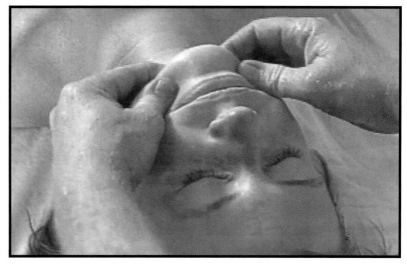

Define the lower jaw with your thumbs and fingers
moving from the midline outward.

Torso Stroke Sequence – Male Client

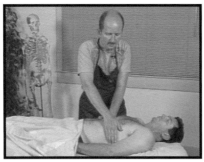

1. Rocking Rib Cage

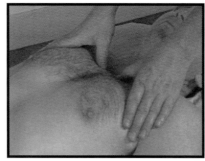

2. Lymphatic Release

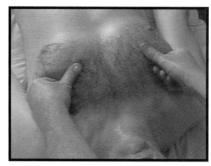

3. Pectoralis Major

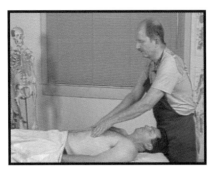

4. Rib Cage

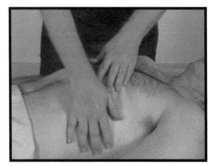

5. Raking Intercostals

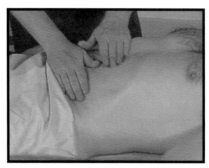

6. Colon Chase

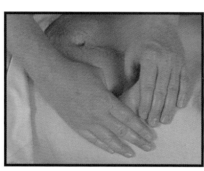

7. Diaphragm Release

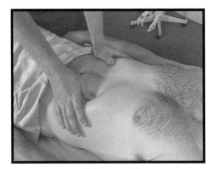

8. Diamond

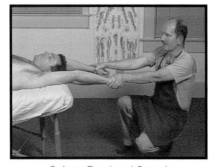

9. Arm Overhead Stretch

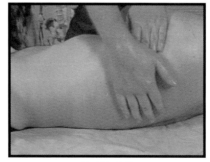

10. Side Lift

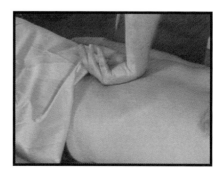

11. Corkscrew

This is only one of many ways to massage the torso.

TMJ Circles

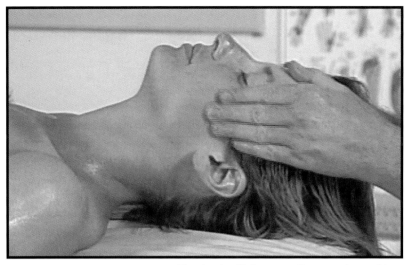 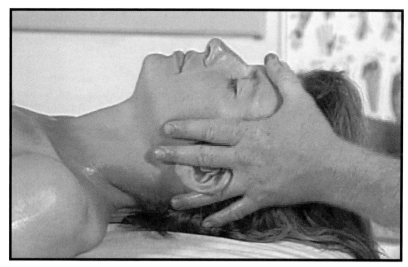

Do circular friction over the masseter and temporalis muscles, first with your fingers then with your whole hand.

Yawn Stretch Stroke

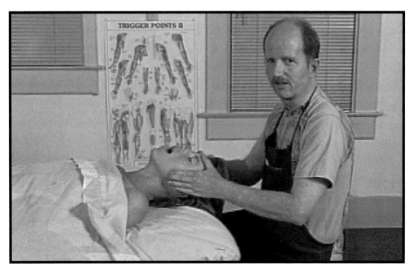 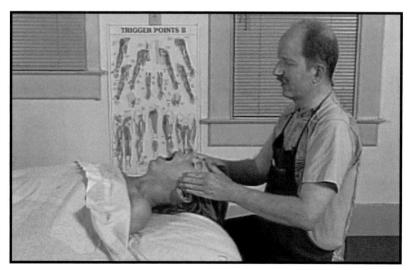

Have client yawn fully as you apply gentle finger pressure into the masseter, enhancing the stretch and working the attachments along the mandible.

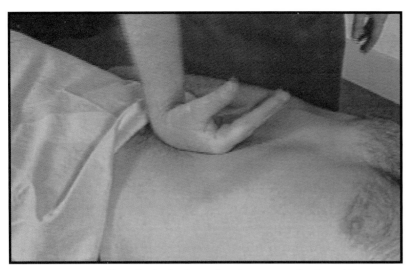 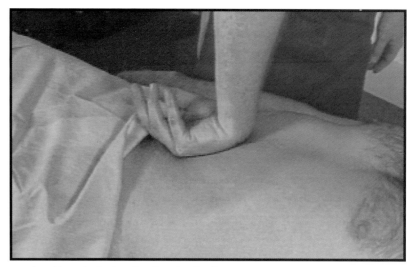

Place the back of your hand over your client's umbilicus and press lightly. Rotate your hand in a clockwise direction, turning it over as necessary.

Forearm Hand Slide

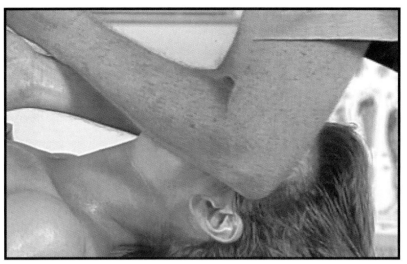
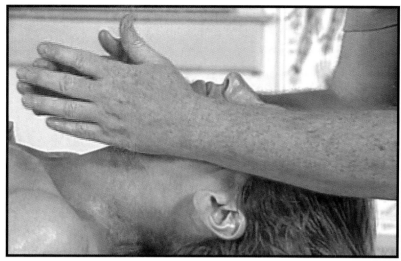

Begin with forearms extended and make a gliding stroke across the face.
Elbows lightly contact face just superior to the mandible, then mold around face with forearms, hands and finally fingertips.

Ear Massage

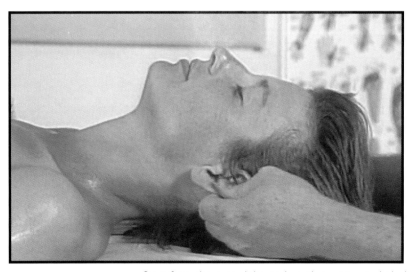
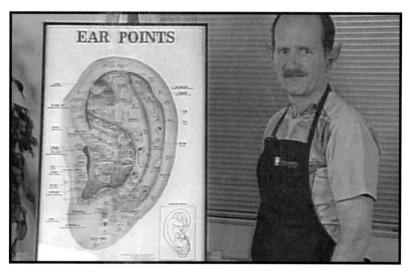

Start from the outer lobe and gently squeeze and pinch moving in towards the inner ear. Take hold of the whole ear and rotate.

Arm Overhead Stretch

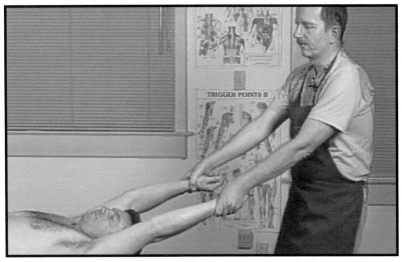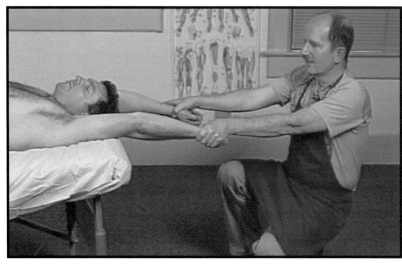

Hold client's arms at wrists. Pull arms over their head and hold as they breathe. As they relax slowly stretch further, staying within their comfort range.
For clients with shoulder restriction, support arms at elbows so humerus is at a tolerable angle and stretch with great sensitivity.

Side Lift

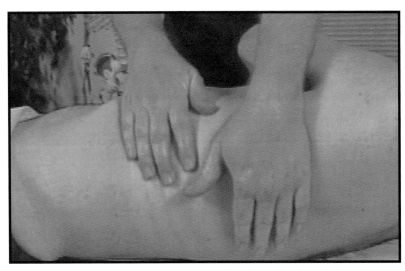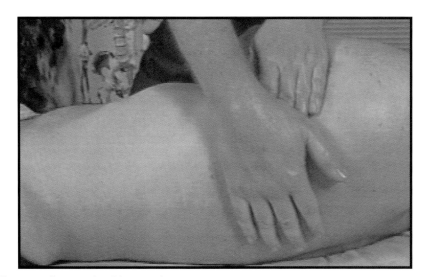

Hand over hand work from iliac crest to shoulder, lifting your client on the side opposite you.

Face Stroke Sequence

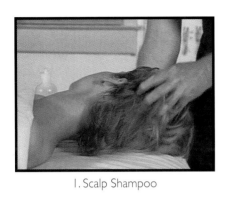
1. Scalp Shampoo

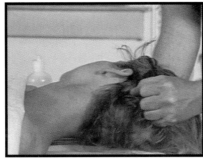
2. Hair Pull Circles

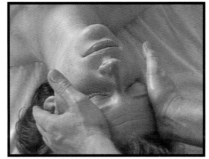
3. Forehead Heel Press

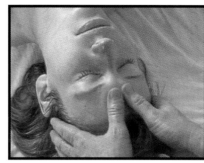
4. Brow Clearing with Thumbs

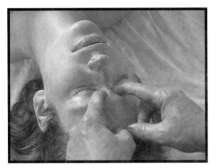
5. Supraorbital Ridge

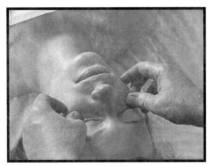
6. Infraorbital Ridge

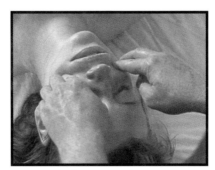
7. Cheekbone Plough

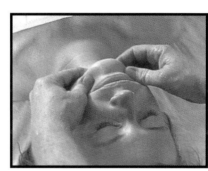
8. Define Maxilla and Mandible

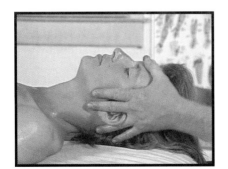
9. TMJ Circles

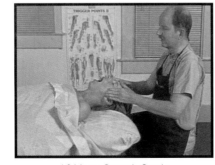
10. Yawn Stretch Stroke

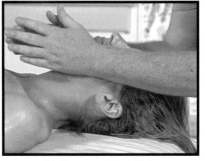
11. Forearm Hand Slide

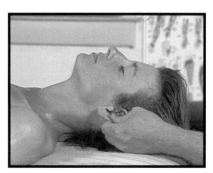
12. Ear Massage

This is only one of many ways to massage the face.

Diamond

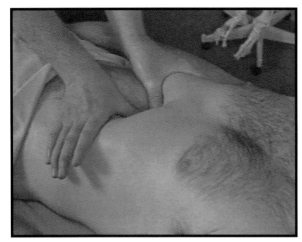

1. Facing superiorly, place thumbs inferior to xyphoid process.

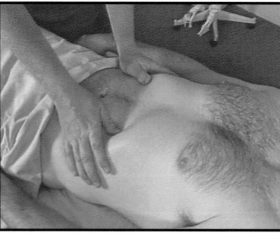

2. Outline ribcage to floating ribs.

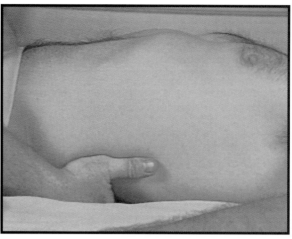

3. Let hands slide under client's back.

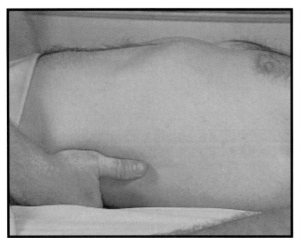

4. Bridge into erector spinae muscles as you pull down to superior border of sacrum.

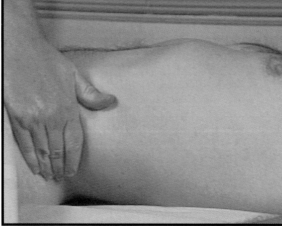

5. Define iliac crest (lifting client's pelvis slightly) to ASIS.

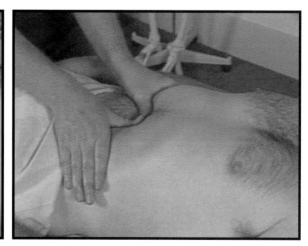

6. Light effleurage to sternum and repeat.

Lift and Pull

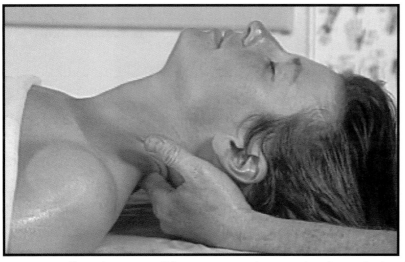
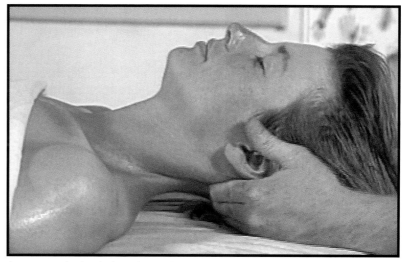

Fingertip pressure sliding up erector spinae muscles of upper back and neck. Elevate neck, accentuating lordosis, and stretch neck gently in superior direction.

Trapezius Stroke

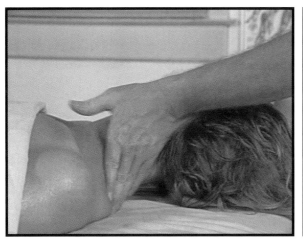
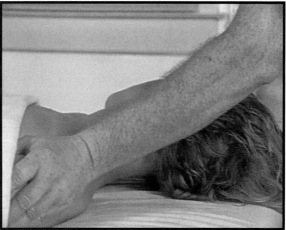
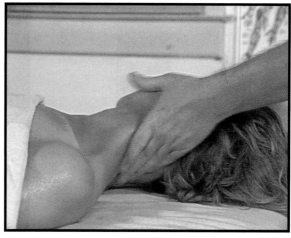

Cradle client's head in one hand with your thumb in front of the ear and your fingers into the occiput, so their head is rotated and laterally flexed.
With your free hand, effleurage from mastoid down neck (keeping posterior to sternocleidomastoid), pivot on shoulder and push inferiorly,
then pull back up with fingertip pressure back to occiput.

Diaphragm Release

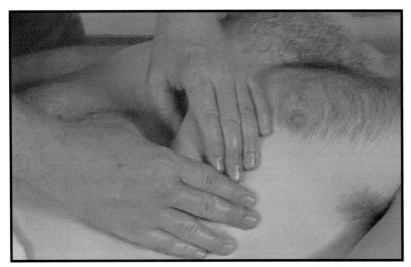 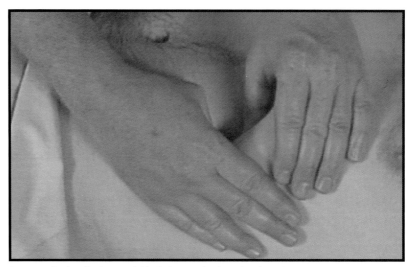

Grasping the lower portion of one side of rib cage, use thumb or finger pressure pressing superiorly towards the diaphragm. Work the entire length of the lower ribcage slowly as client breathes deeply; exercising care to avoid pressure on the floating ribs. Client may have knees elevated.

Levator Scapulae, Supraspinatus

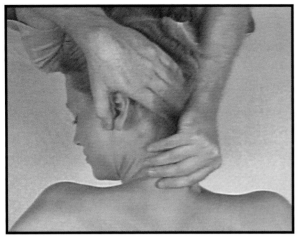 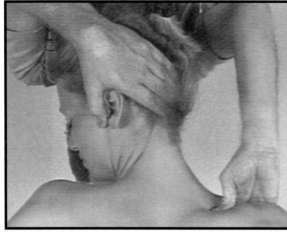 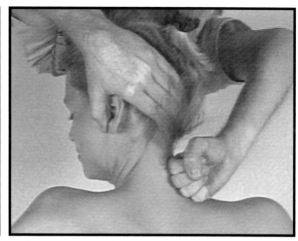

Deep pressure into levator scapulae and supraspinatus muscles with thumbs or knuckles. (Shown from underneath the table).

Occiput Circles

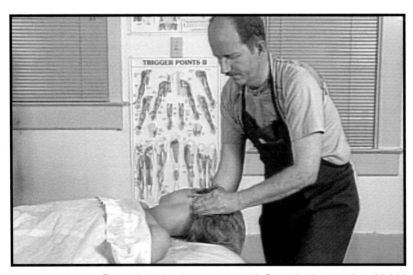 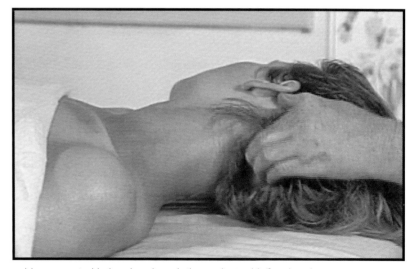

Deep slow circular pressure with fingertips into occiput. Hold head rotated to one side, supported in hand, and work the occiput with free hand.

Raking Intercostals

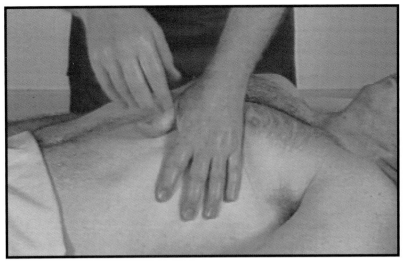 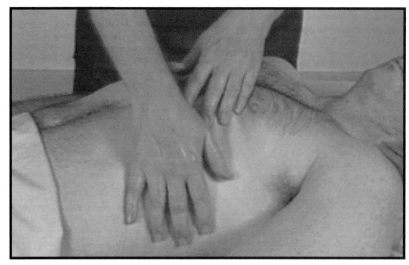

Work on opposite side of table with fingertip pressure between ribs.
This may be done repetitively hand over hand, slowly and carefully, or very slowly and specifically with deeper pressure.

Colon Chase

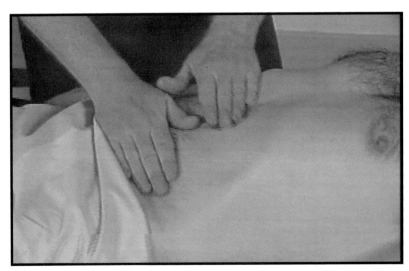 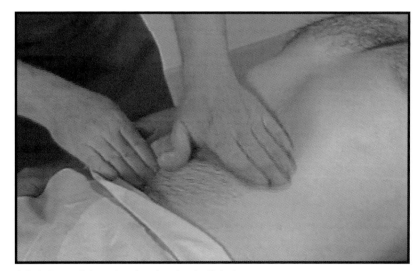

Effleurage with both hands clockwise over colon. One hand makes full circles and the other hand makes half circles.

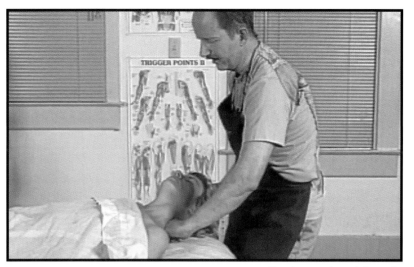 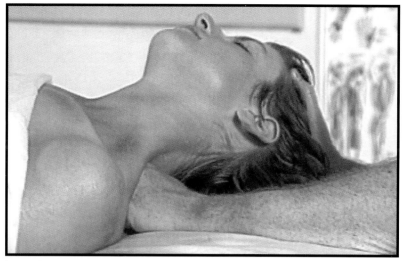

Gently stretch neck laterally so that the ear is drawn closer to the shoulder
while stabilizing client's opposite shoulder with your other hand. Stroke with knuckles from occiput to shoulder.

Pectoralis Major

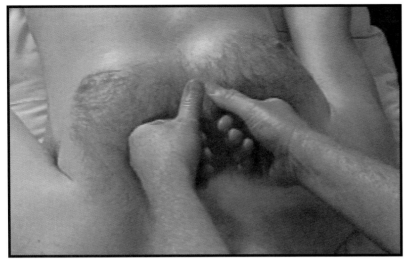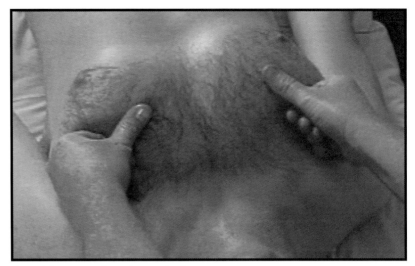

Work with knuckles moving from the sternum toward the insertion of the pectoralis major on the humerus.

Rib Cage

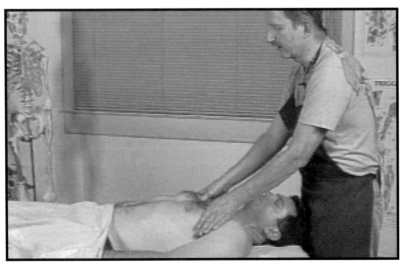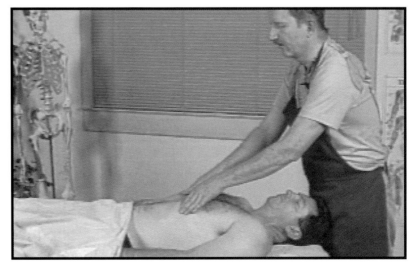

Use thumbs or fingers to work intercostal spaces going laterally from the sternum.

Neck Stroke Sequence

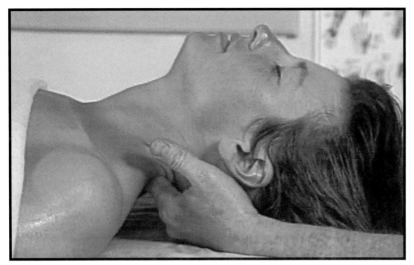

1. Lift and Pull

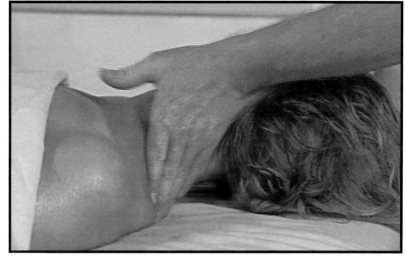

2. Trapezius Stroke

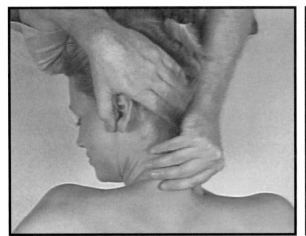

3. Levator Scapulae and Supraspinatus

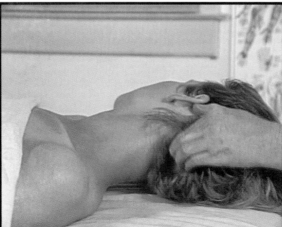

4. Occiput Circles

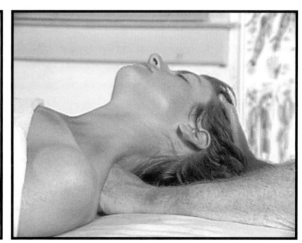

5. Lateral Flexion

This is only one of many ways to massage the neck.

Rocking the Rib Cage

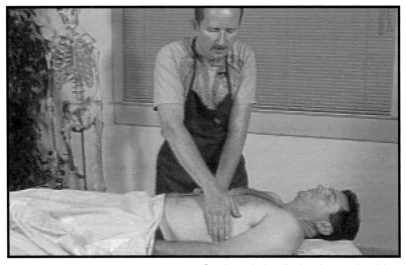
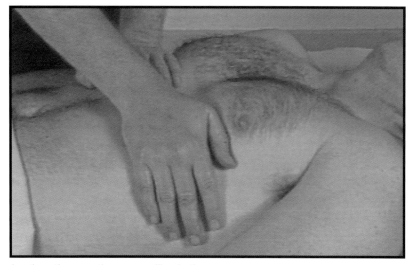

Gently rock the ribs by alternately raising one side and lowering the other, creating a wave-like rhythm.
Notice mobility and restrictions. Use open palm, with pressure exerted between the ribs.

Sternum Release and Lymphatic Clearing

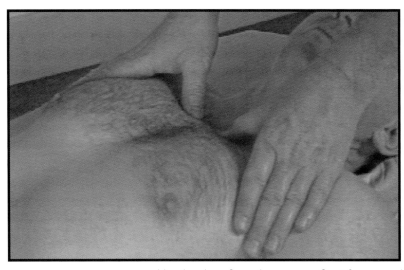
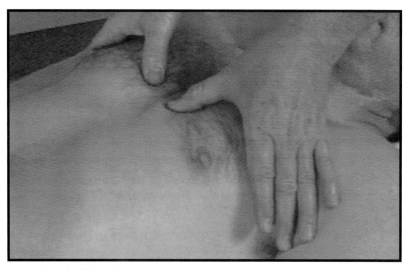

Use thumb or fingertip pressure. Start from superior border of sternum and work all the rib attachments on both sides.
Pressing into, pulling away from, or tiny circles directly on the sternal border are all effective.

Long Stroke

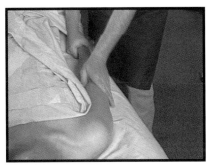

1. Hold wrist with inside hand and effleurage up arm with outside hand.

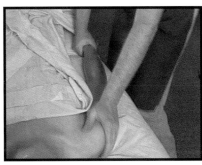

2. Hook around deltoid.

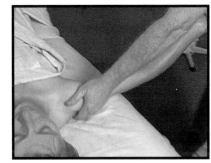

3. Bring arm overhead, while

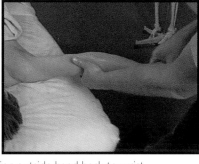

4. gliding outside hand back to wrist

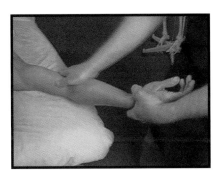

5. Switch hands - hold wrist with outside hand and effleurage with inside hand to axilla.

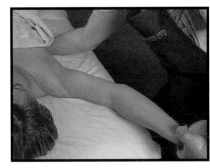

6. Continue effelurage to low back.

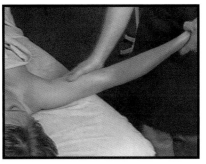

7. Bring arm back down to side, while

8. gliding inside hand back to wrist.

Torso Stroke Sequence – Female Client

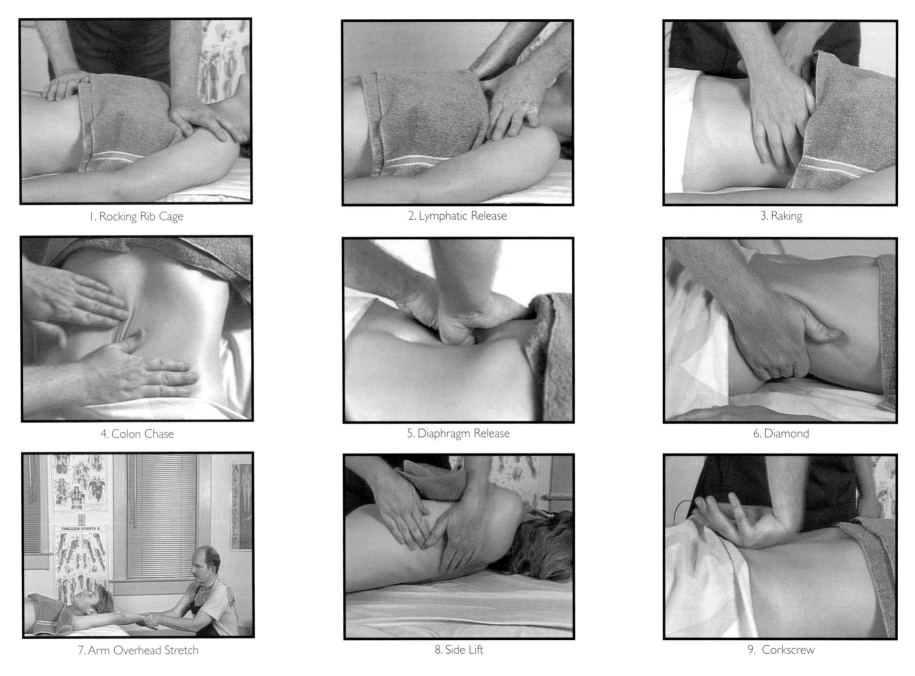

1. Rocking Rib Cage

2. Lymphatic Release

3. Raking

4. Colon Chase

5. Diaphragm Release

6. Diamond

7. Arm Overhead Stretch

8. Side Lift

9. Corkscrew

This is only one of many ways to massage the torso.

Wrist Articulation

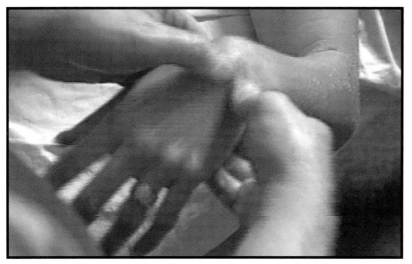
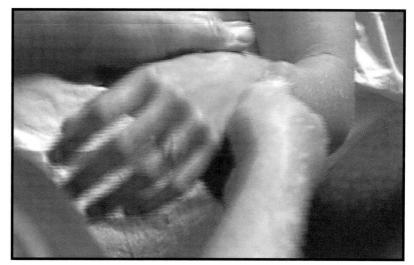

Thumbs on posterior of wrist, fingers completing hold, explore movement between carpal bones with a gentle flicking motion.

Metacarpal Grooves

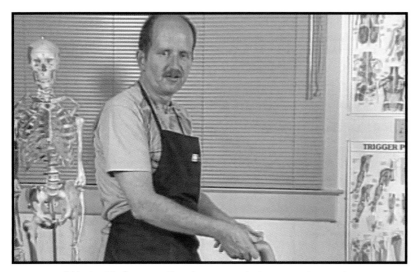

Work with finger or thumb pressure between metacarpals.

Articulate Fingers

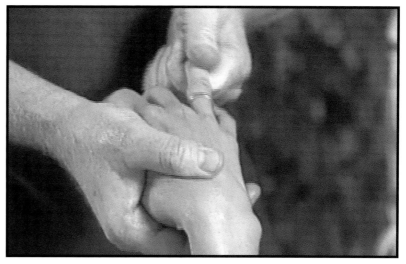

Support client's hand at metacarpals while working fingers with your other hand.

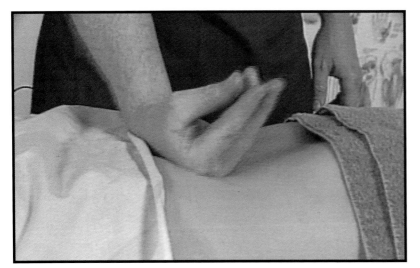 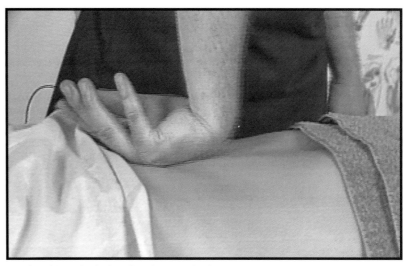

Place the back of your hand over your client's umbilicus and press lightly. Rotate your hand in a clockwise direction, turning it over as necessary.

Palm Stretch Stroke

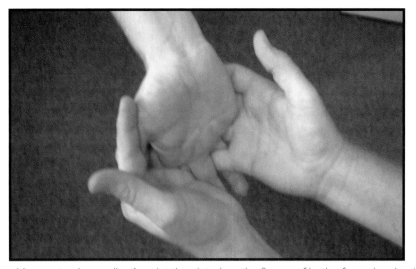
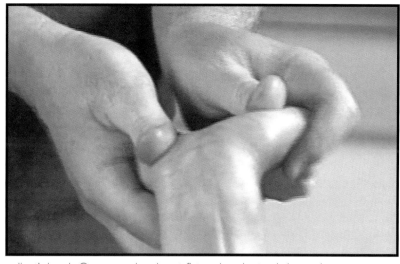

Hyperextend your client's wrist, then interlace the fingers of both of your hands with fingers of your client's hand. Open your hands out flat and apply steady increasing pressure to client's hand causing the wrist to be extended into stretch. Ask for feedback from client when to stop. Hold for a few seconds at end of stretch, then release stretch some but keep fingers interlaced while massaging client's palm with your thumbs.

Wrist Circumduction

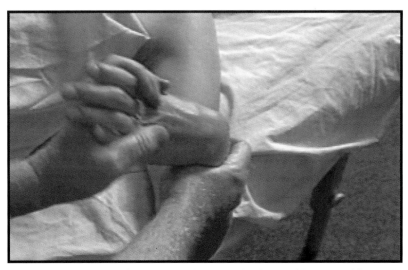
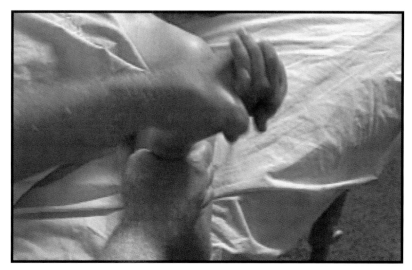

Support client's arm at distal end of forearm while moving the client's hand around in as wide an arc as possible with your other hand.

Arm Overhead Stretch

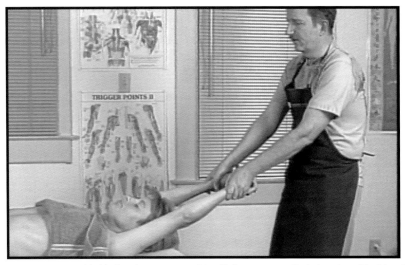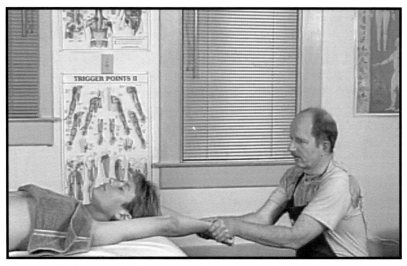

Hold client's arms at wrists. Pull arms over their head and hold as they breathe. As they relax slowly stretch further, staying within their comfort range.
For clients with shoulder restriction, support arms at elbows so humerus is at a tolerable angle and stretch with great sensitivity.

Side Lift

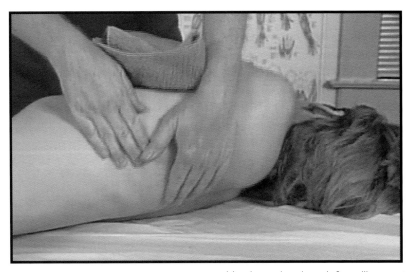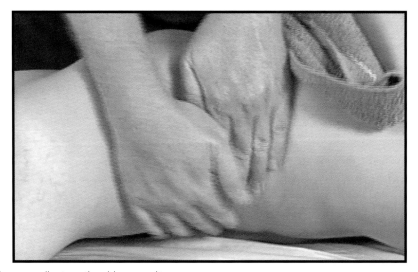

Hand over hand work from iliac crest to shoulder, lifting your client on the side opposite you.

Ghost Hand

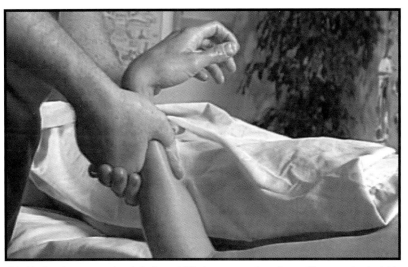

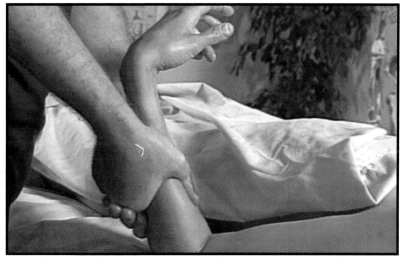

Hold client's arm so that it is flexed 90 degrees at the elbow (forearm is straight up and elbow is supported on table). Make a ring around the forearm just proximal to client's wrist and stroke firmly to their elbow giving deep effleurage to extensors and flexors. Alternating thumbs may also be employed.

Arm Cradle

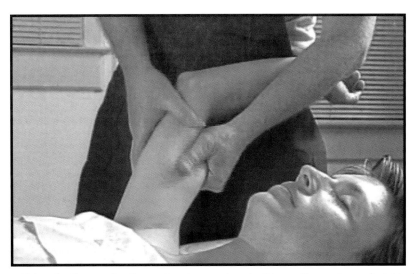

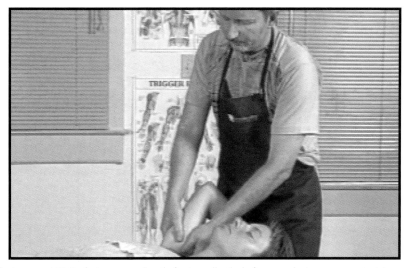

Raise client's arm directly overhead, or as close to this position as is comfortable, flexing elbow 90 degrees. While facing your client's feet cradle their forearm between your inside elbow and the crest of your ilium. Perform petrissage, effleurage and wringing into biceps, triceps, and deltoid.

Diamond

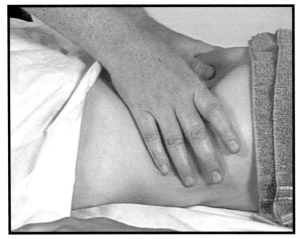

1. Facing superiorly, place thumbs inferior to xyphoid process.

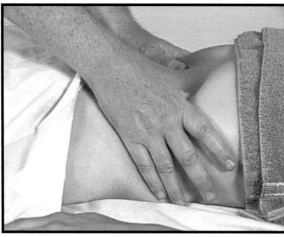

2. Outline ribcage to floating ribs.

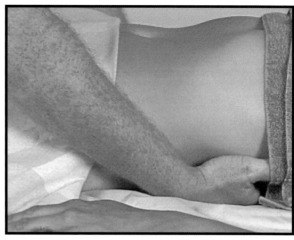

3. Let hands slide under client's back.

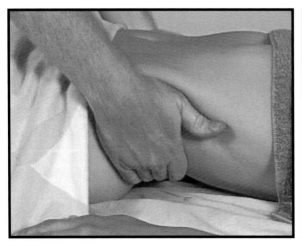

4. Bridge into erector spinae muscles as you pull down to superior border of sacrum.

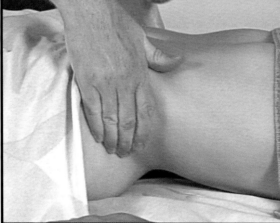

5. Define iliac crest (lifting client's pelvis slightly) to ASIS.

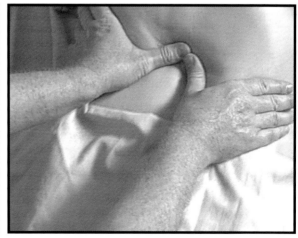

6. Light effleurage to sternum and repeat.

Deltoid, Rhomboids

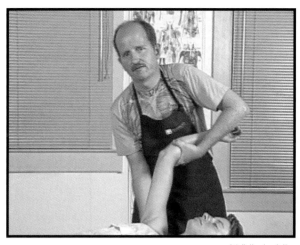
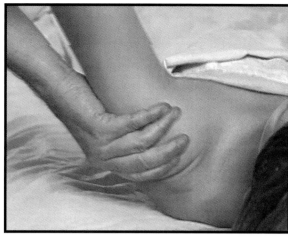
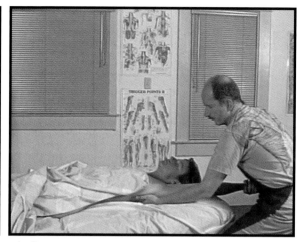

While holding forearm with inside hand, hook outside hand around deltoid and effleurage.
Slide outside hand under shoulder to medial border of scapula and hook into rhomboids while stretching arm overhead.

Shake Arm to Side

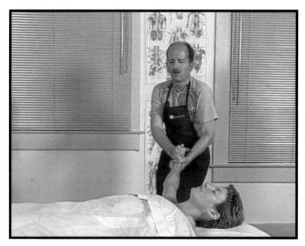
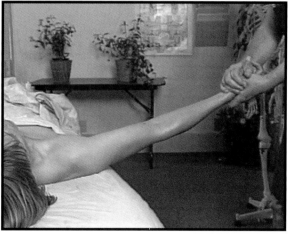
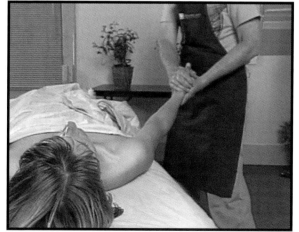

Holding hand at wrist, shake arm as you give traction to it and bring it back to client's side.

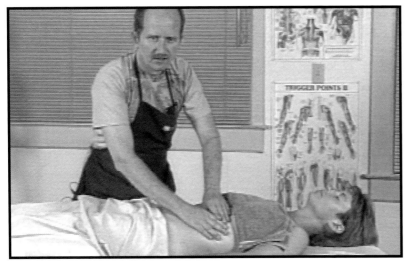 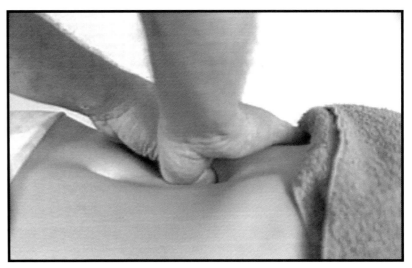

Grasping the lower portion of one side of rib cage, use thumb or finger pressure pressing superiorly towards the diaphragm. Work the entire length of the lower ribcage slowly as client breathes deeply; exercising care to avoid pressure on the floating ribs. Client may have knees elevated.

Bridging into Scapula

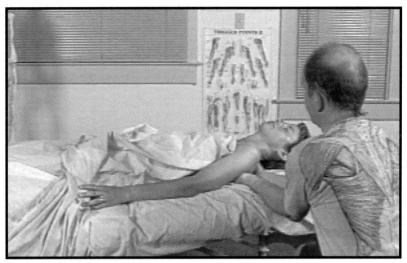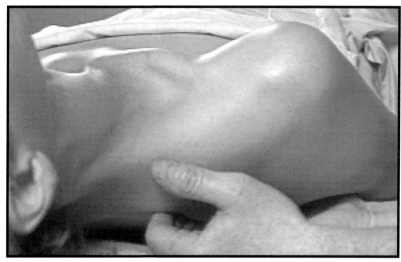

Elevate shoulder, slide your outside hand under scapula, creating a bridge with your fingertips. Allow weight of shoulder to gently stretch and give pressure to scapula attachments. Place both hands under scapula with an 8 finger bridge, move fingers, gently stretching scapula attachments.

Arm Stretch

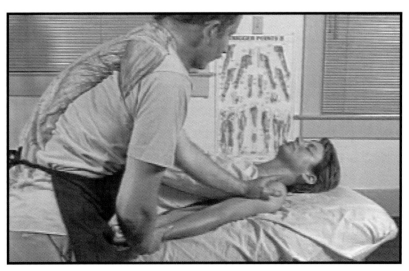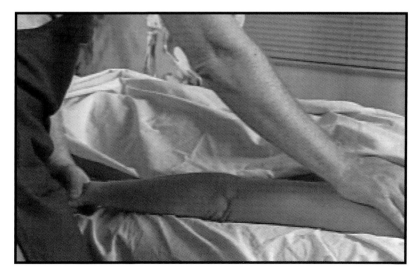

With heel of hand press shoulder joint superiorly while pulling client's hand inferiorly with other hand.

Raking Intercostals

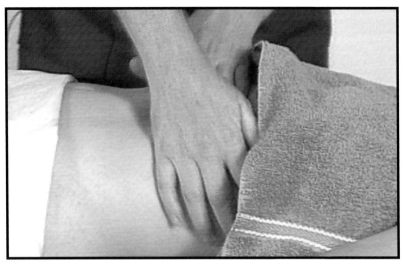 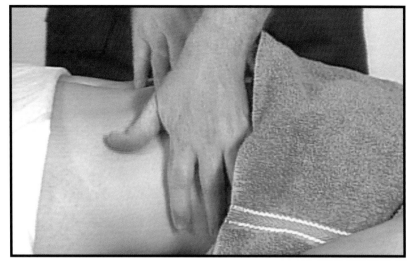

Work on opposite side of table with fingertip pressure between ribs. This may be done repetitively hand over hand, slowly and carefully, or very slowly and specifically with deeper pressure. Do not work over breast tissue.

Colon Chase

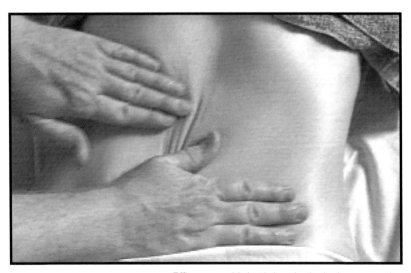 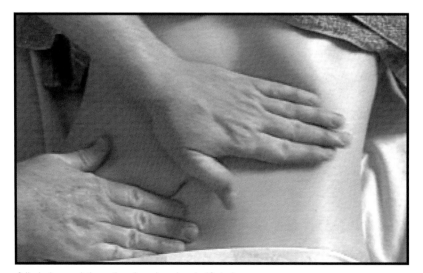

Effleurage with both hands clockwise over colon. One hand makes full circles and the other hand makes half circles.

Arm Stroke Sequence

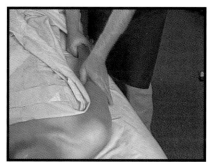
1. Long Stroke

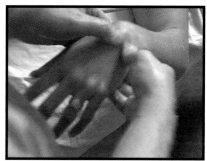
2. Wrist Articulation

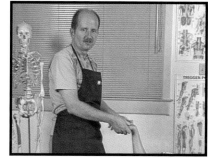
3. Metacarpal Grooves

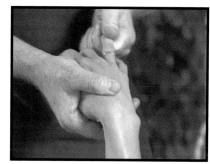
4. Articulate Fingers

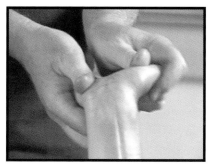
5. Palm Stretch

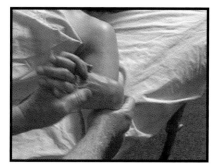
6. Wrist Circumduction

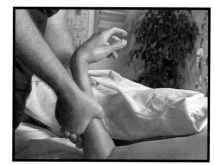
7. Ghost Hand

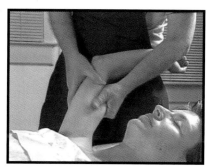
8. Arm Cradle

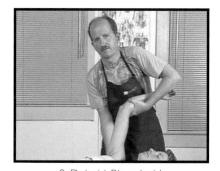
9. Deltoid, Rhomboids

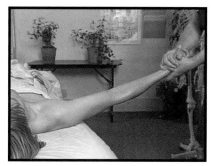
10. Shake Arm to Side

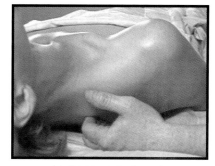
11. Bridging into Scapula

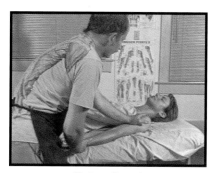
12. Arm Stretch

This is only one of many ways to massage the arm.

Rocking the Rib Cage

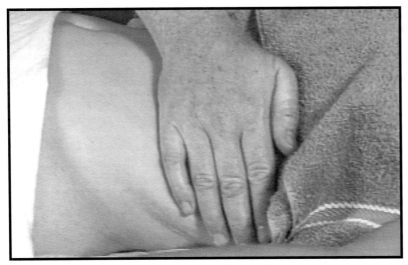
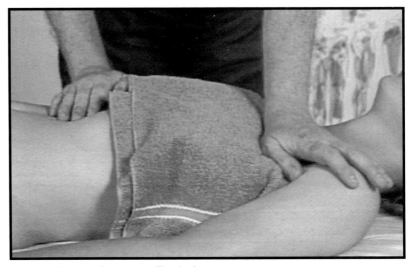

Gently rock the ribs by alternately raising one side and lowering the other, creating a wave-like rhythm.
Notice mobility and restrictions. Use open palm, with pressure exerted between the ribs.

Sternum Release and Lymphatic Clearing

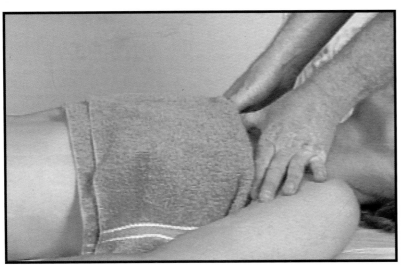
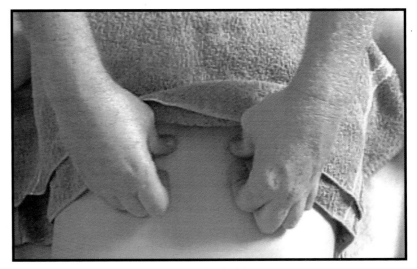

Use thumb or fingertip pressure. Start from superior border of sternum and work all the rib attachments on both sides.
Pressing into, pulling away from, or tiny circles directly on the sternal border are all effective.